An Atlas of
PSORIASIS
Second edition

THE ENCYCLOPEDIA OF VISUAL MEDICINE SERIES

An Atlas of
PSORIASIS
Second edition

Lionel Fry MD FRCP

Professor Emeritus of Dermatology
Imperial College
London, UK

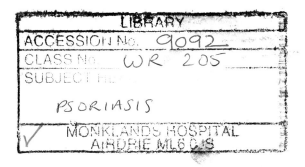
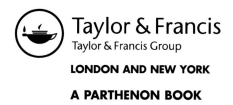

Taylor & Francis
Taylor & Francis Group

LONDON AND NEW YORK

A PARTHENON BOOK

© 2004 Taylor & Francis, an imprint of the Taylor & Francis Group

First published in the United Kingdom in 2004
by Taylor & Francis,
an imprint of the Taylor & Francis Group,
11 New Fetter Lane,
London EC4P 4EE

Tel.:   +44 (0) 20 7583 9855
Fax.:   +44 (0) 20 7842 2298
Website: www.tandf.co.uk

British Library Cataloguing in Publication Data

Data available on application

Library of Congress Cataloging-in-Publication Data

Data available on application

ISBN 1-84214-237-2

Distributed in North and South America by

Taylor & Francis
2000 NW Corporate Blvd
Boca Raton, FL 33431, USA

Within Continental USA
Tel.: 800 272 7737; Fax.: 800 374 3401
Outside Continental USA
Tel.: 561 994 0555; Fax.: 561 361 6018
E-mail: orders@crcpress.com

Distributed in the rest of the world by
Thomson Publishing Services
Cheriton House
North Way
Andover, Hampshire SP10 5BE, UK
Tel.: +44 (0) 1264 332424
E-mail: salesorder.tandf@thomsonpublishingservices.co.uk

Composition by Parthenon Publishing
Printed and bound by T.G. Hostench, S.A., Spain

Contents

Introduction

Psoriasis is a common skin disorder with a world-wide distribution but is more common in the Caucasians of the western world. So far, the disease has retained its secrets of what actually causes the psoriatic lesion; whilst considerable advances have been made in its management in recent years, there is no absolute cure, and no simple, safe and invariably effective treatment. The first description of psoriasis is credited to Celsus (25 BC–AD 45), but Hippocrates (460–375 BC) probably did see psoriasis, under his heading of 'scaly eruptions', and called them lopoi (from lepo, to scale). Galen (AD 133–200) was the first to use the word 'psoriasis' (taken from the Greek word psora – the itch). However, from the description of the rash given by Galen, he was probably describing seborrheic eczema (scaling and itching of the eyelids). However, the nosology of so-called seborrheic eczema is now open to question as it is indistinguishable from so-called seborrheic psoriasis. Thus, it is possible that this entity is a variant of psoriasis, so Galen may have been correct. Celsus, in his description of the disease as it is recognized today, described the disease under the term 'impetigo' (from impeto, to attack). Thus, from the outset, it would appear that the wrong names were given to skin disorders which are recognized today. Until the end of the eighteenth century, psoriasis and leprosy were grouped together, and psoriatics often faced the same fate as lepers in the fourteenth century, being burnt at the stake. The clinical patterns of psoriasis, as we know them today, were first described by Willan at the beginning of the nineteenth century and the disorder was separated from leprosy in 1841 by the Austrian dermatologist Hebra.

Lionel Fry

1

Epidemiology and histology

The incidence of psoriasis has been estimated by census studies and postal questionnaires, and the reliability of some of the studies is open to question. The highest reported incidences have been in Denmark (2.9%) and the Faroe Isles (2.8%)[1]. The average for Northern Europe (including the UK) has been given as 2.0%, and Northern Europe is generally considered as having the highest incidence. The incidence in the USA is 1.4%. There appears to be a higher incidence in East, as opposed to West, Africans, and this may explain the low incidence in African-Americans. The Arabs have been reported to have an incidence similar to that of the Northern Europeans. There is a low incidence in the Asians of China and the Far East, the incidence in China being reported as 0.37%. The results for the Indian subcontinent have been variable: some studies give a lower incidence than in Europeans, whilst others have reported a similar incidence. The disease is said to be non-existent in the Native Americans, and the Aborigines from Samoa. However, the reliability of most of these studies is questionable, apart from those carried out in Northern Europe. The general impression is that the highest incidence is in Europeans, and the lowest in Asians from the East.

The two characteristic histological features of psoriasis are epidermal hyperplasia and an inflammatory cell infiltrate in both the dermis and the epidermis. In the initial stages, there is slight epidermal hyperplasia with thickening of the rete ridges. The epidermal cells increase in size and there is enlargement of the nucleus, dilatation of the intercellular spaces and infiltration with lymphocytes and macrophages. At a later stage, there is infiltration with polymorpho-nuclear leukocytes. As the lesion progresses, the epidermal cells show lack of differentiation and further increase in size and number. The granular layer begins to disappear and abnormal parakeratosis appears. This is loosely bound keratin within which are found degenerative neutrophils. Exudation of neutrophils into the epidermis leads to accumulation of these cells in the upper epidermis, where small micro-abscesses form. In the dermis, there is enlargement and tortuosity of the capillaries, which migrate upwards into the dermal papillae. There is an infiltrate of lymphocytes, particularly

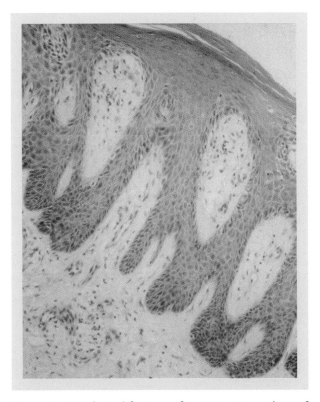

Figure 1 Histological features of psoriasis. Hyperplasia of the epidermis. Poorly formed granular layer, hyperkeratosis and parakeratosis of the stratum corneum. Collection of neutrophils in the epidermis

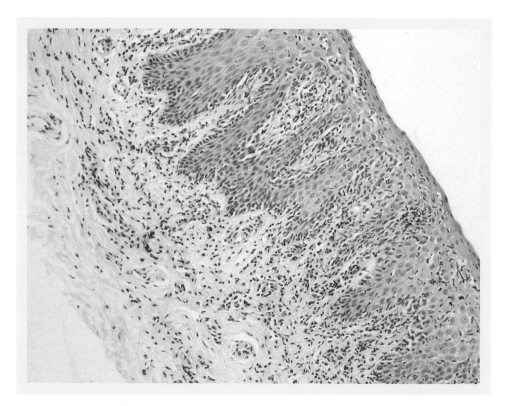

Figure 2 Histological features of psoriasis. Heavy lymphocytic infiltrate in the dermis

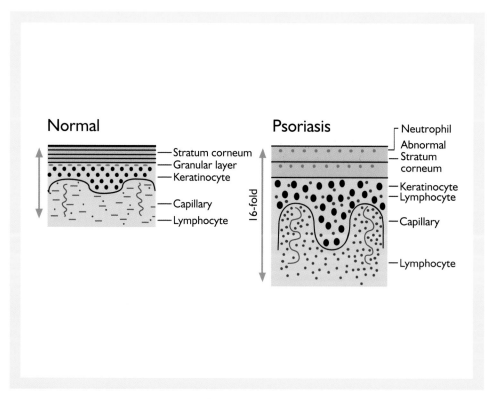

Figure 3 Diagrammatic comparison of normal skin with established psoriasis. There is a 16-fold increase in the thickness of the skin in psoriasis

around dermal capillaries in the deep papillary network, and, to a lesser extent, of macrophages and occasional neutrophils.

In established psoriasis (Figures 1–3), there is elongation and thickening of the rete ridges, elongation and edema of the dermal papillae, absent, or a poorly formed, granular layer, parakeratosis, micro-abscess in the epidermis, enlargement of the capillaries and a mainly lymphocyte infiltrate around the subpapillary vessels. The basal layer shows an increase of mitotic figures. The re-arrangement of the basement membrane configuration results in its considerable lengthening, due to the elongation of the rete ridges. This feature is characteristic of hyperplasia of the epidermal cells. In fact, other features, such as elongation and dilatation of the capillary loops, and swelling and elongation of the dermal papillae, are also adjustments that have to be made in the architecture of the skin to sustain the increase in cell numbers and their increased metabolic activity. The absent granular layer and abnormal keratin layer (parakeratosis) are probably due to a maturation defect of the rapidly proliferating keratinocytes. Thus, it is possible that the fault in psoriasis is one of rapidly dividing epidermal cells and the histological features are secondary to this proliferation. What stimulates the epidermal cells to proliferate is discussed in the section on etiology. However, there is some evidence that the hyperproliferation of the keratinocytes is secondary to a maturation defect of these cells[2].

In pustular psoriasis, the neutrophils accumulate in greater numbers within the epidermis to form a macro-abscess. What initiates this rare process is unknown, but it is probably related to an increase in neutrophil chemotactic factors.

2

Prognosis

It is difficult to give a true incidence of the remission rate of psoriasis, as a large proportion of individuals with slight clinical involvement do not attend dermatological clinics, or even any doctor. Therefore, most studies of the natural history are based on results from specialist centers where the more severe forms of the disease are seen. Psoriasis tends to run a variable course; it may have spontaneous remissions which are temporary or permanent, therapy-induced remissions, which again may be temporary or permanent, or it may run a persistent course. The interval of time between the episodes of psoriasis, in those who have remissions, may vary from a few months to several years.

In reported studies, the figures for permanent remission are not favorable. In one study[3] of patients followed up for 21 years (but in which only 54% were available for continuous assessment), 71% had persistent lesions 13% were free of the disease and 16% had intermittent lesions. In a study of 30 000 inhabitants of the Faroe Isles over a 20-year period[1], similar results were obtained: at follow-up after 5

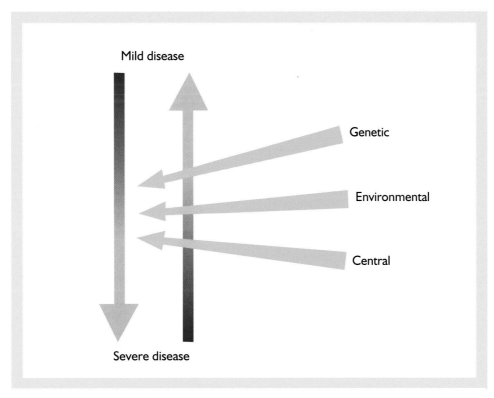

Figure 4 Factors affecting disease activity

years 17%, after 10 years 14%, and after 20 years 6% were disease-free. However, 48% of the patients had a remission during the 20-year follow-up. Another study, of 5000 patients in the USA[4], reported that 39% of the patients had a remission which varied from 1 to 84 years. It is difficult to give a firm prognosis to patients with psoriasis because of the variable course. However, a number of clinical features tend to imply a poor outlook; these include early onset, that is under the age of 10 years, extensive and persistent disease, and disease which begins on the face and trunk. Psoriasis which begins after the age of 25 tends to have a better prognosis. Erythrodermic and generalized pustular psoriasis have a poor prognosis, with the disease tending to be severe and persistent. Localized pustular psoriasis is a persistent disorder with over two-thirds of patients having the disease for more than 10 years[5]. Guttate psoriasis usually has a good prognosis, particularly in children. The disease tends to resolve after 3 months.

However in two reports on the follow-up of guttate psoriasis one[6] found that two-thirds of patients went on to develop chronic plaque disease while the other[7] found only one-third had chronic plaque psoriasis after 10 years.

The prognosis is related to what may be described as 'disease activity' (Figure 4). There appear to be central factors controlling psoriasis as well as local ones. The more active the disease, the poorer the prognosis. Active disease is difficult to clear and relapses quickly after cessation of treatment. The biological factors controlling 'disease activity' are not yet known. However, clinically active disease is associated with appearance of new lesions and extensive involvement. Disease which is inactive undergoes spontaneous resolution. Disease activity may change in time within an individual patient and this adds to the uncertainty in trying to give a firm prognosis.

3

Genetics

FAMILY STUDIES

It has been known for many years that psoriasis has a hereditary basis, as it was noted that the disease tended to run in families. The early observations supporting an inherited factor were derived from family studies. One of the earliest was in a closed community in a small town in Germany, conducted over a 30-year period. It was found at the beginning of the study that 34% of patients with psoriasis had a positive family history; 5 years later this number had increased to 39%, and at the end of the 30 years it was 56%[8]. Some studies of families with psoriasis through three and four generations strongly support the concept of Mendelian dominance with incomplete penetration, as every affected child had an affected parent. However, other family studies through a similar number of generations did not find that all affected individuals with psoriasis had an affected parent, and asymptomatic carriers were assumed. These latter studies considered that the inheritance was autosomal recessive with 90% penetration. The more recent studies have suggested that psoriasis is a polygenic disorder, i.e. several genes are involved in the pathogenesis. In addition, the etiology of psoriasis is multifactorial, i.e. with environmental as well as genetic factors interacting to produce the manifestations of the disease. This interaction and the involvement of several genes is now referred to as a complex multifactorial disease.

CENSUS STUDIES

There have been two classical census studies: one in the Faroe Isles which studied 30 000 individuals[1], and another in Sweden which covered 40 000[9]. In the latter, it was found that 6.4% of relatives of patients with psoriasis were affected, compared to 1.96% of the general population. In the study in the closed community in the Faroe Isles, 91% of patients with psoriasis had a family history. This high figure was probably due to the special circumstances of the closed community. Analysis of the data in these two census studies supports the current concept that in psoriasis there is multifactorial inheritance and that simple monogenic types of inheritance are now excluded.

TWIN STUDIES

These strongly support the role of inheritance in psoriasis, as the concordance in monozygotic twins is 65–70%, whilst that for dizygotic twins is 15–20%. Twin studies have also shown that the clinical type of psoriasis, age of onset, the course and severity are determined to a large extent by genetic factors.

HUMAN LEUKOCYTE ANTIGENS

Early studies of the class I human leukocyte antigens (HLA) showed an association of psoriasis with B13, B17 and B37. Recently, B57 has also been found to be associated with psoriasis. However, the strongest association of the class I HLA is with Cw6 and the association with the B antigens is thought to be due to linkage disequilibrium with Cw6[10]. The strongest association is with the Cw*0602 allele. Three ancestral haplotypes (Cw*0602-B13, Cw*0602-B37 and Cw*0602-B57) have an increased risk of developing psoriasis, the highest being associated with Cw*0602-B57 and the lowest with Cw*0602-B37.

The highest incidence of Cw6 in patients with psoriasis is in Caucasians, where studies have shown the incidence varying between 36 and 84%, the average being 60–65%. The incidence of Cw6 in non-psoriatic Caucasian patients is 10–15%. The frequency of Cw6 is considerably lower in Asian patients with psoriasis; a study in Japan reported an occurrence of 26%[11] and in Chinese patients, 17%[12]. However, because the incidence of Cw6 in the Far Eastern Asian populations is very low (1–2%), the relative risk for developing psoriasis in Cw6 patients is greater than in Europeans (25% in Japanese and 20% in Chinese). The relative risk for psoriasis is 8.9% in Europeans if patients are Cw6 heterozygous and 23% if patients are homozygous for Cw6[13]. However, it should be remembered that only 10% of individuals who carry Cw6 actually develop psoriasis, so that other factors are necessary for expression of the disease.

Clinical features of psoriasis show a relationship to Cw6[14,15]. This HLA antigen is associated with the early onset of the disease, guttate eruptions, a positive family history and increased severity of psoriasis. However, this is not an absolute association and patients may have these features if they are Cw6 negative. There is controversy as to whether Cw6 is a gene for psoriasis or whether the gene is in linkage disequilibrium with Cw6 and is close to the HLA-C locus. The fact that Cw6 is in linkage disequilibrium with the B13, B37 and B57 HLA antigens and the observation that there are different relative risks for psoriasis with the three different haplotypes Cw*0602-B13, Cw*0602-B37 and Cw*0602-B57 suggests that the gene is not likely to be HLA-Cw6.

The class II antigens DR7 and DR4 are also significantly increased in psoriasis and the strongest association is with DR7[16]. The incidence in Caucasians with psoriasis is approximately 60% compared to the frequency in the general population of 9–10% with a relative risk of 7.0 for psoriasis.

The association between class II HLA and the clinical features has been lacking until recently. A recent study, however, has suggested that DR15 is associated with late onset, no history of guttate episodes and relatively mild disease[17]. These features are the opposite of those associated with Cw6. DR15 or a gene in linkage disequilibrium with DR15 may therefore be acting as a modifying factor in the psoriatic process.

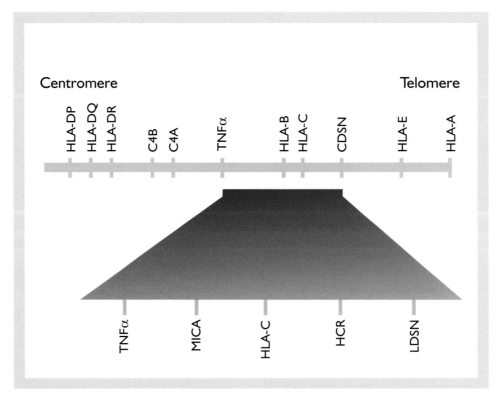

Figure 5 MHC region on chromosone 6 with expanded area for possible susceptibility genes, (CDSN, cormeodesmosin, HCR, and MICA). This diagram is not to scale

CHROMOSOME LOCI AND POSSIBLE GENES

Several genome scans have been performed in psoriasis. These have not always employed the same methods, i.e. some have looked at multiplex families and others at 'sib-pairs'. In addition, these studies have also looked at different ethnic groups. The loci reported in chronological order have been 17q25 (American), 4q34 (mainly Irish), 6p21.3 (British), 1q21 (Italian), 3q (Swedish), 19q13 (German), 1p (British) and 4q31 (Chinese).

Not all these loci have been confirmed in subsequent studies but this may be due to variation in ethnicity. The locus which has been confirmed most often is that on 6p21.3. This locus includes HLA Cw6. However, when this locus is fine mapped using both polymorphic microsatellite markers and single nucleotide polymorphisms (SNPs), there has been no agreement as to the exact region within the 6p21.3 locus that is associated with psoriasis. Most studies have not found linkage to Cw6 itself but to regions both centromeric and telomeric to Cw6.

Within the locus 6p21.3, certain candidate genes have been suggested and investigated[18,19]. These genes include corneodesmosin, MICA, TNFα, and Cw6 itself (Figure 5). Thus, at present, despite the confirmation by several groups of linkage between psoriasis and 6p21.3, no gene has been confirmed. It may be relevant that no difference has been found in the sequence of Cw6 in psoriasis patients and in non-affected individuals.

No gene mutation has been found in the other loci linked to psoriasis, although very recently, a mutation in SLC9ARI has been reported in the 17q25 locus[20]. This gene is concerned with the transport of ions across cell membranes and immune synapse formation in T cells with the transcription factor RUNX 1. Targets for RUNX proteins are yet to be elucidated. Confirmation of the mutation in the SLC 9 ARI gene is awaited. Interestingly, in the locus on chromosome 3q it has been reported in Swedish families that the gene SLC12A8 associates with psoriasis, although no structural abnormality in this gene has so far been reported[21].

4

Etiology

ENVIRONMENTAL TRIGGERS

Although there is undoubtedly a genetic component to the development of psoriasis, environmental factors are also important, and may trigger the disease.

PHYSICAL TRAUMA

In approximately one-third of patients with psoriasis, trauma to the skin will result in the development of psoriatic lesions at the site of trauma. This phenomenon was first noted by a physician named Koebner in 1872, and it is now known as the Koebner phenomenon. The nature of the injury is immaterial (Koebner himself described the simultaneous development of psoriasis, in an individual, at the sites of a horsefly bite, a tattoo, bacterial infection and excoriations from horse riding). Although one-third of patients with psoriasis develop lesions after injury to the skin (Koebner-positive), two-thirds do not (Koebner-negative). The Koebner phenomenon is 'all or nothing', that is patients who are Koebner-positive at one site are positive everywhere, and those who are negative are negative at all sites. This implies that there is a central factor which influences the development of psoriasis. However, patients may transfer from a state of Koebner positivity to negativity, and vice versa; thus, the central factor influencing the development of psoriasis is variable. It has been shown that the injury inducing psoriasis in a Koebner-positive patient must cause epidermal damage. This injury is likely to produce a cytokine cascade, which triggers psoriasis (see section on pathogenesis). The inhibitory factor which stops the development of psoriasis is likely to be part of an immune response and is possibly related to regulatory T lymphocytes.

A recently described phenomenon is the 'reverse Koebner'. In this situation, removal of part of a psoriatic plaque, by shaving through the plaque in the upper dermis, results in that area being replaced by normal-looking skin unaffected by psoriasis. The reverse Koebner and true Koebner are mutually exclusive, that is patients who are Koebner-positive are positive at all sites and cannot exhibit the reverse Koebner, whilst those who show the reverse Koebner do so at all sites and the Koebner phenomenon cannot be induced.

INFECTIONS

The organism most commonly associated with psoriasis is the β-hemolytic streptococcus. The original observations were made some 50 years ago when it was noted that tonsillitis often preceded the first appearance of psoriasis[22]. It was subsequently shown that, in patients with psoriasis, there was a significantly higher incidence of a positive streptococcal agglutination test, compared to patients with other skin diseases. The clinical association of guttate psoriasis and streptococcal infections is much stronger than that of similar infections and plaque psoriasis. Either one or more of the following are present in over half of the patients with guttate psoriasis: history of a sore throat; approximately 2 weeks before the eruption, a positive throat swab for β-hemolytic streptococcus; and a raised antistreptolysin titer. Confirmation of a streptococcal infection in all patients with guttate psoriasis may be difficult because the patients are usually seen a few weeks after the infection, and the antistreptolysin test is not always positive after infection. It has been shown that guttate psoriasis is induced not only by group A β-hemolytic streptococci but also by groups C and G[23]. However, no particular M serotype has been found to be associated with psoriasis[24].

The role of streptococcal organisms in chronic plaque psoriasis is less certain compared to the guttate form. However, it has been found that there is a higher incidence of positive throat cultures for β-hemolytic streptococci and raised ASO titers compared to a control population[25].

Patients with chronic plaque psoriasis may also develop an acute flare-up of guttate-type papules following a streptococcal throat infection and there may also be an associated increase in size of the chronic plaques of psoriasis. It has also been reported that there is a higher incidence of sore throats in patients with chronic plaque psoriasis compared to a control group[26]. Thus, there is both actual and suggestive evidence of an increase of streptococcal throat infections in chronic plaque psoriasis.

One of the reasons for failure to demonstrate the streptococcal organisms by throat swabs is that the organisms have the ability to become intracellular and in this location are not detected by routine throat swabs. In addition, once the streptococci become intracellular in the tonsillar epithelial cells, they are not eradicated by penicillin, which cannot penetrate the cell walls. This also allows the streptococcus to persist in the tonsils and be a reservoir for streptococcal antigens, which may be responsible for maintaining the disease (see pathogenesis). Further evidence for a role for the streptococcus in psoriasis is the demonstration that circulating and skin T cells show an increased proliferative response and gamma interferon (IFN)-γ production to streptococcal antigens[27].

Other organisms that have been implicated as playing an etiological role in psoriasis, are *Staphylococcus aureus* and *Candida albicans*[28] and *Pityrosporum orbiculare*[29]. Viral infections may also play a role in the etiology of psoriasis, as the eruption appears, or the pre-existing disease is aggravated, by an influenza-type illness. Whether this is specific for the virus or whether this is due to associated bacterial infections, which cannot be demonstrated by routine bacteriological tests, has yet to be determined. Finally, psoriasis may appear at the sites of chicken pox or herpes zoster, but this is likely to represent a Koebner reaction, rather than a specific effect of the virus.

STRESS

There is no doubt that, in patients with the genetic predisposition for psoriasis, stress may precipitate psoriasis and aggravate existing disease. However, the widely held view by patients that psoriasis is due to 'nerves' is not correct. The proportion of patients with psoriasis in whom stress plays an important role as a trigger is difficult to estimate, because of the problems of defining stress and because various stressful situations affect individuals differently, depending on their personality. Studies on the grade of neuroticism in patients with psoriasis have not shown any difference compared to a control group.

How stress induces or aggravates psoriasis is not known. Stress has effects on hormones, and the autonomic nervous and immune systems. There is now accumulating evidence that the immune system is involved in disease expression and this may lead to alteration in the homeostatic mechanisms which control epidermal proliferation, the hallmark of psoriasis. It has also been recently shown that neuropeptides secreted by nerve endings in psoriasis may influence immune cells in the skin and keratinocyte function. This could be another mechanism by which stress may affects psoriasis.

DRUGS

Certain drugs, notably lithium, β-blockers, antimalarials (chloroquin, hydroxychloroquin and quinacrine) and non-steroidal anti-inflammatory drugs (NSAIDs), have been reported to aggravate psoriasis. How these different drugs with different chemical structures can have the same effect is difficult to explain; they may affect the psoriatic process at different stages but with the same results. Steroids, both systemic and topical, have a beneficial effect on psoriasis, but withdrawal of systemic steroids (and occasionally potent topical steroids) may result in flare-up of psoriasis, and, for this reason, systemic steroids tend not to be used in the treatment of psoriasis.

HYPOCALCEMIA

It is an interesting observation that the very rare condition of hypocalcemia aggravates psoriasis. This observation may be of importance in unraveling the pathogenetic pathway of the psoriatic process, particularly as vitamin D, both orally and topically, improves psoriasis.

ALCOHOL

There has long been a reported association between psoriasis and a high intake of alcohol. Originally this was attributed to patients taking alcohol in an attempt to alleviate their feelings of frustration and anxiety/depression because of their psoriasis.

However, more recent studies have shown a deleterious effect of alcohol on the psoriatic process, but the mechanism has to be elucidated.

CLIMATE

Psoriasis tends to improve in warm climates and to become worse in cold ones. This seems to be independent of the effects of ultraviolet light. This effect of climate on psoriasis may partly explain the high incidence of the disease in the Northern European countries.

5

Pathogenesis

IMMUNOPATHOLOGY

Psoriasis is characterized by epidermal and dermal features. In the epidermis, there is proliferation and impaired maturation of the epidermal cells (keratinocytes) with a resulting defect in keratinization and failure to produce a normal skin barrier (Figures 1–3). In the dermis, there is a lymphocytic infiltrate and an increase in the capillary network in the dermal papillae (Figures 1–3). Until the 1980s, the primary fault in psoriasis was thought to be one of uncontrolled keratinocyte proliferation. However, over the past 20 years, it has been shown that this keratinocyte proliferation is mediated by T lymphocytes[30].

In the early stages of guttate psoriasis, there is an influx and activation of CD4 T cells into the dermis and epidermis and these T cells are in close apposition to the dendritic processes of the antigen-presenting cells (APCs) (Figure 6). During resolution of guttate psoriasis, there is an influx and activation of CD8 cells into the epidermis. In this stage of the

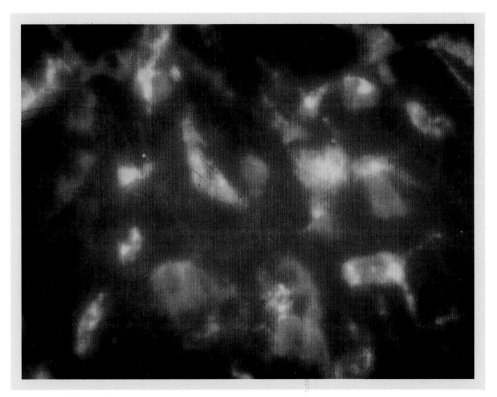

Figure 6 CD4 lymphocytes (red) in close apposition to the dendritic processes (green) of the antigen-presenting cells (Langerhans cells) in the initiation of guttate psoriasis

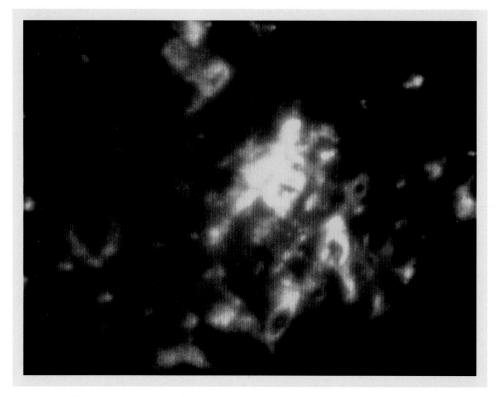

Figure 7 CD8 lymphocytes (red) in close apposition to the dendritic processes (green) of antigen-presenting cells in the resolution of guttate psoriasis

disease, the CD8 cells are found in close apposition to the dendritic processes of the APCs (Figure 7). In guttate psoriasis, it is likely that the CD4 cells are the effector cells inducing the hyperproliferation, whilst the CD8 cells are the regulatory cells inducing a remission of the psoriatic process.

In chronic plaque psoriasis, there is an influx of mainly CD4 cells in the dermis, but in the epidermis there are both activated CD4 and CD8 cells. It has been assumed that the CD4 cells are the primary effector cells and the CD8 cells play a regulatory role. More recently, it has been suggested that the CD8 cells in chronic plaque psoriasis may, in fact, be effector cells[31] (see below).

ANTIGEN-PRESENTING CELLS

There is an increase in the total number and number of activated APCs in both the dermis and the epidermis, implying increased antigen presentation by these cells to T lymphocytes (the nature of the antigen is discussed below).

The antigen induces maturation of the APCs and migration of these cells to the regional lymph nodes where the APCs interact with naïve T cells, resulting in T cell activation. This process requires at least two signals: the first is the antigen in the MHC molecule of the APC reacting with the T cell receptor (TCR) of the lymphocyte; and the second is the co-stimulating signals from the APC to the T cell (Figure 8). Subsequent to the interaction between the APCs and T cells, the latter proliferate and become memory T cells and enter the circulation. When they enter the skin and meet the antigen they will become activated and produce cytokines, which will stimulate keratinocyte proliferation.

CYTOKINES

It was suggested in the mid-1980s that cytokines produced by activated T cells induced the activation and proliferation of the keratinocytes. The cytokine production by T lymphocytes has been subdivided into Th1 and Th2 profiles. The Th1 cytokines are IFNγ, interleukin (IL)-2, tumor necrosis factor (TNF)-α and transforming growth factor (TGF)-β; and Th2 cytokines are IL-4, IL-5, IL-10 and IL-13. In psoriasis, the cytokines most commonly detected are

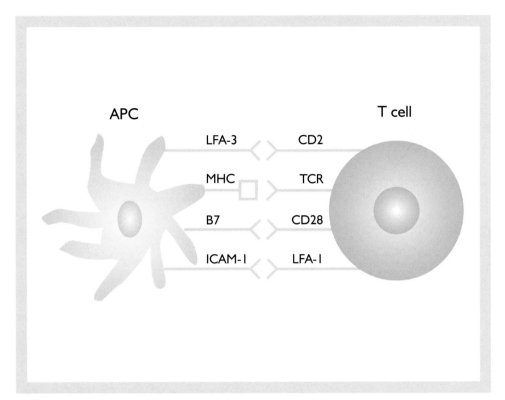

Figure 8 Activation of T lymphocyte by antigen presentation from APC. The antigen is presented by specific MHC molecule to specific T cell receptor. Co-stimulating signals are also required between the two cells; these may be via LFA-3 to CD2; B7 to CD28 or ICAM-1 to LFA-1. LFA-3, lymphocyte function antigen-3; ICAM-1, intercellular adhesion molecule-1; LFA-1, lymphocyte functional antigen-1

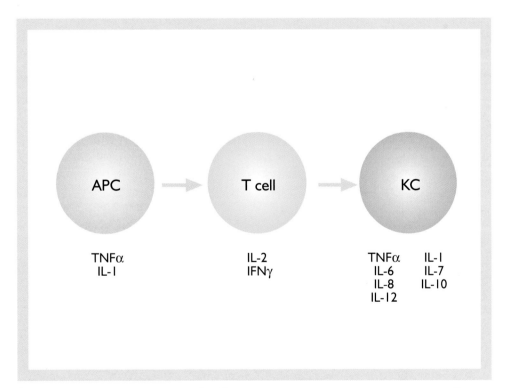

Figure 9 Cytokine production of cells in psoriasis. APC, antigen presenting cell; KC, keratinocyte

IFNγ and IL-2, i.e. a Th1 cytokine profile. No IL-4 is found in psoriasis, but IL-5 has been detected; therefore, in psoriasis, it is possible there may be a distinct subset of T cells secreting both Th1 and Th2 cytokines. The specific cytokines responsible for proliferation of keratinocytes have not been established, but IFNγ is necessary for the development of psoriasis, because neutralization of this cytokine with specific antibody blocked the mitogenic activity.

Keratinocytes once activated have been shown to produce a large number of cytokines, which may induce further proliferation of these cells and have other proinflammatory and immunomodulatory effects. The cytokines identified are IL-1, IL-6, IL-7, IL-8, IL-10, IL-12 and TNFα (Figure 9). IL-8, which is abundant in psoriatic scale, is strongly chemoattractive for neutrophils and probably accounts for the micro-abscesses that are found in the upper epidermis in psoriasis.

The central role for T lymphocytes in psoriasis is supported by the observation that psoriasis clears with systemic cyclosporin and tacrolimus, whose primary action is to inhibit IL-2 production by activated T cells. In addition, a CD4 monoclonal antibody clears psoriasis, supporting the hypothesis that these cells play a fundamental role in both inducing and maintaining the psoriatic process.

NATURE OF THE ANTIGEN

The trigger most commonly associated with psoriasis is Streptococcus pyogenes. Throat infection with this organism can induce guttate psoriasis and there is also some evidence that it is associated with chronic plaque disease. The S. pyogenes organism secretes a number of extracellular products including pyrogenic exotoxins, hemolysins and enzymes. A role for exotoxins has been suggested in psoriasis and, in addition, the cellular proteins may also be involved (Figure 10).

STREPTOCOCCAL EXOTOXINS

There are several streptococcal exotoxins, which act as superantigens. They include streptococcal exotoxins (SPE-A, -C, -F, -X) and S. pyogenes mitogen-2 (SPM-2). These substances have the ability to activate a large number of T cells and not one specific clone. Superantigens bind to the outer aspect of the MHC class II molecule and are not restricted to a

particular class II allele, as are specific peptides. Once the superantigen is bound to the MHC molecule it then binds to the TCR via its Vβ region (Figure 11). There are 24 different Vβ families and the different toxins bind to specific Vβ families. Because the toxins are not restricted to a particular MHC class II allele or a specific TCR they have the ability to activate a large number of T cells. This mechanism has been implicated in guttate psoriasis, as it has been found that there was a significant increase in Vβ2, and, to a lesser extent, Vβ 5.1 T cells in the skin lesions but not in the blood, which suggests a selective recruitment of these cells into the skin[32]. Confirmation that this influx and activations of the T cells was due to a superantigen, came when sequence analysis of the TCR Vβ2 genes revealed extensive junctional region diversity rather than oligoclonality of the TCR, which would be seen with a conventional antigen[33]. An increase in particular Vβ families has also been found in chronic plaque psoriasis[32] and in exacerbations of chronic plaque psoriasis thought to be associated with S. aureus and C. albicans. Both these organisms secrete superantigens. Thus, a role for bacterial superantigens does appear likely at least, in guttate psoriasis, in acute flares of chronic plaque psoriasis and possibly even in stable chronic plaque psoriasis.

CELLULAR STREPTOCOCCAL PROTEINS

The cell wall proteins include M proteins, T proteins, receptors for IgA and IgG and the cell wall and membrane proteins themselves. M and T proteins are fibrillar structures anchored to the cell wall and membrane (Figure 10).

The M protein is often considered to be the major virulence factor of the organism. It is composed of a proximal conserved region (C-terminus) and a distal variable one (N-terminus). The variable part of the M protein confers the organism's serotype, of which there are now over 80.

The cell wall itself is composed mainly of a structure called peptidoglycan, which is composed of polysaccharides linked by peptide bridges. The structure of the cell membrane and its antigenic components are yet to be determined.

The analysis of the TCR in chronic plaque psoriasis has shown a significant proportion to be oligoclonal, suggesting that the T cell response in this form of the disease is by a specific antigen and TCR (Figure 8). A number of streptococcal antigens have

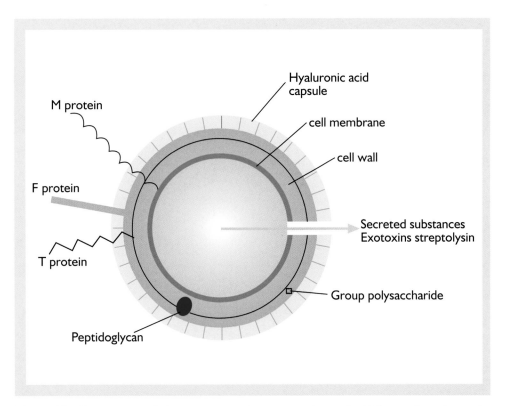

Figure 10 Components of the streptococcal organism some of which may be relevant in psoriasis

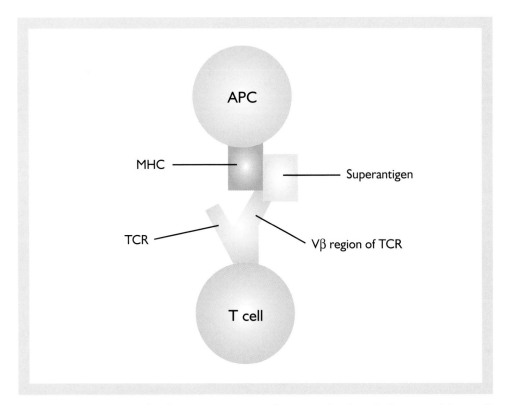

Figure 11 Superantigen binding to outer aspect of MHC molecule and Vβ region of the T cell receptor (TCR)

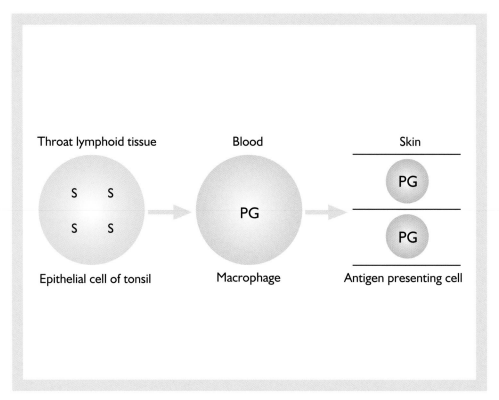

Figure 12 Possible pathway of peptidoglycan (PG) from intracellular streptococcus (S) in the throat

been suggested as being those maintaining psoriasis. The two main ones have been M protein peptides and other cell wall antigens.

EVIDENCE FOR M PROTEIN BEING THE ANTIGEN IN PSORIASIS

M proteins show amino acid sequence homology with a number of human proteins including tropomysin, myosin and certain keratins. Cross reactivity of M protein with antigens, including those in synovium and brain, and heat shock proteins, have also been demonstrated. Peripheral blood mononuclear leukocytes (PBML) and CD4 T cells from patients with both guttate and chronic plaque psoriasis have shown increased proliferative responses and increased IFNγ production when stimulated with whole streptococcal antigens. Subsequently, it was shown that T cells isolated from the blood had increased IFNγ production to peptides sharing homology for M proteins and keratin 17[34,35]. It was suggested that there is cross reactivity between M protein and keratin 17. Thus, T cells primed to react to streptococcal M protein would also react to keratin 17. The latter is not present in normal skin (apart from hair follicles) but is present in psoriatic skin. The hypothesis put forward is that T cells, specific for certain M protein peptides could initiate chronic plaque psoriasis and, once the disease was produced in the skin, keratin 17 would be formed. Peptides homologous for M protein and keratin 17 would be formed and maintain the disease. If this is correct then psoriasis could be called an autoimmune disorder.

EVIDENCE FOR OTHER CELL WALL AND MEMBRANE PEPTIDES BEING THE ANTIGEN IN PSORIASIS

In more recent studies, CD4 T cells isolated from psoriatic skin did not show an increased proliferative response or IFNγ production to M protein[36,37], but there was a response to other cell wall and membrane extracts. It was also shown that the CD4 T cells in psoriatic skin showed these increased responses to streptococcal peptidoglycan. In support of streptococcal peptidoglycan being a possible antigen in psoriasis was the observation that there was a significant increase in APCs and macrophages containing peptidoglycan in psoriasis lesions (B.S. Baker, personal communication). The source of this streptococcal antigen may be persistent intracellular organisms in the tonsils or other lymphoid tissue in the throat (Figure 12). There is even the possibility that streptococcal organisms or their components are present in the skin, but in what form is speculative.

ARE THE EFFECTOR T CELLS IN PSORIASIS CD4 OR CD8?

Activated CD4 T cells are present in the dermis of both guttate and chronic plaque psoriasis. The epidermal activated CD4 T cells are characteristic of guttate psoriasis and are not present in resolving lesions. This suggests that the CD4 cells are the effectors. However, in chronic plaque psoriasis, there are both activated CD4 and CD8 T cells. In addition, oligoclonality of the TCR was demonstrated in the CD8+ T cells and, as these cells persisted over a period of time, it was suggested that these cells may be the effectors[38]. In addition, because of the high incidence of the HLA Cw6 in psoriasis, which is a class I antigen, it has been suggested that Cw6 plays an active role in presenting antigens to the CD8 cells[31]. It has also been found that both CD8 and CD4 cells in the epidermis produce IFNγ when stimulated with whole streptococcal antigens. However, when uninvolved skin from a psoriasis individual is transplanted onto SC1D mice (these animals lack immune cells), injection of activated CD4 but not CD8 cells will induce psoriasis, implying that CD4 cells are the effectors[39]. It is conceivable that both CD4 and CD8 T cells have an effector role in psoriasis. In addition, both CD4 and CD8 cells could be regulatory under different conditions. There is no doubt that central factors influencing immune responses are operative in psoriasis (although their exact nature has yet to be elucidated), but they could well determine the behavior of T cells.

HOW DO THE T CELLS ENTER THE SKIN?

T cells enter and leave the skin all the time as part of immune surveillance. In psoriasis there is an excessive influx of these cells into the skin. For memory T cells, (CD45RO+) to gain entry into the skin, they

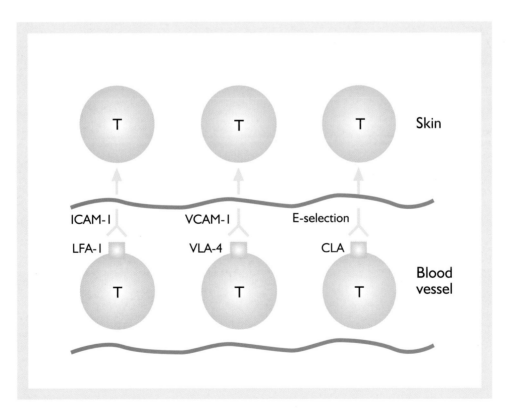

Figure 13 Antigens on T cells bind to adhesion molecules on the endothelial cells to gain entry into the skin. ICAM-1, Intercellular adhesion molecule-1; LFA-1, Lymphocyte functional antigen-1; VCAM-1, Vascular cell adhesion molecule; VLA-4, Very late antigen; CLA, Cutaneous lymphocyte antigen

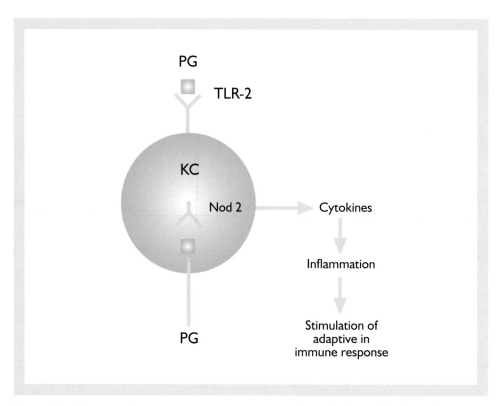

Figure 14 The innate immune response to streptococcal peptidoglycan. Possible role in psoriasis. PG, peptidoglycan; KC, keratinocyte; TLR-2, Toll like receptor-2

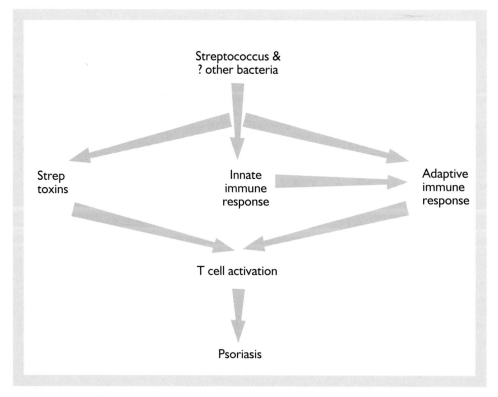

Figure 15 Possible pathways for induction of psoriasis by bacterial micro-organisms

must express the lymphocyte function-associated antigen LFA-1 and very late antigen VLA-4, which bind to adhesion molecules in the endothelial cell wall, i.e. intercellular adhesion molecule (ICAM)-1, for LFA-1 and vascular adhesion molecule (VCAM)-1 for VLA-4. In addition, for the T cells to enter the skin, they have to express cutaneous lymphocyte antigen (CLA). Normally, only a few memory T cells express CLA. However, superantigens, including streptococcal ones, induce CLA expression, so this may be a further role of streptococcal organisms in psoriasis. The CLA antigen binds to E-selectin on the endothelial cell wall. Thus, a set of antigens and receptors on the T cell and endothelial cells are necessary for the T cell to enter the skin (Figure 13). The expression of the receptors on the endothelial cell is up-regulated by the cytokines released by APCs, T cells and keratinocytes, so the process is self-perpetuating. Once inside the skin, the T cells will migrate, owing to interaction with other cells and extracellular components under the influence of chemokines and cytokines.

THE INNATE IMMUNE SYSTEM

The innate immune system is the most ancient system of defense against pathogenic organisms in animals. The system does not rely on the recognition of specific peptides of organisms, as does the more sophisticated so-called adaptive immune system. The innate immune system relies on a set of receptors on cell surfaces that recognize highly conserved microbial motifs (pathogen-associated molecular patterns (PAMPs)). The receptors on the mammalian cells are known as Toll-like receptors (TLRs) and eight of the ten recognize bacterial motifs. TLR-2 recognizes peptidoglycan from Gram-positive bacteria. TLR-2 is expressed by keratinocytes in both normal skin and that with psoriatic lesions. In normal skin, it is found predominately in the basal layer whilst in psoriasis, it is found throughout the keratinocyte layer. More recently, two intracellular molecules (Nod 1 and Nod 2) have been found in epithelial cells and macrophages and they are also concerned with recognition of bacterial molecules. Nod 2 has been shown to recognize peptidoglycan of Gram-positive organisms. Once the bacterial motifs are recognized by the cell-surface and intracellular receptors, the cells will produce cytokines, which in advanced mammals will attract lymphocytes and APCs into the tissue, and the so-called adaptive immune response will follow (Figure 14).

Because psoriasis is triggered by the streptococcus and the fact that streptococcal peptidoglycan is found in increased quantity in psoriatic skin, it is possible that peptidoglycan may stimulate both the innate and, subsequently, the adaptive immune system in psoriasis (Figure 15). In support of this hypothesis is the observation that CD4 T cells in psoriasis show increased proliferative responses and IFNγ production to streptococcal peptidoglycan (B.S. Baker, personal communication).

Recently a mutation in the Nod 2 gene has been found in patients with Crohn's disease. There is a known association between psoriasis and Crohn's disease, in that patients with Crohn's disease have a higher incidence of psoriasis and vice versa. Thus, a defect in the innate immune system and the response to bacteria may be relevant to the etiology of both diseases.

6

Clinical features

AGE OF ONSET

Psoriasis may begin at any age, but it is rare under the age of 10 years. It is most likely to appear first between the ages of 15 and 30 years. In some 60% of patients, the disease will begin before the age of 30. The incidence of presentation then gradually falls with age, but psoriasis may first appear in the eighth and ninth decades. As a general rule, the earlier the age of onset the worse the prognosis.

SEX PREDILECTION

Psoriasis affects males and females equally.

MORPHOLOGY

The classical lesion of psoriasis is a well demarcated raised red plaque with a white scaly surface (Figure 16). However, the color of a psoriatic plaque depends on the thickness of the scale and whether it is adherent or loosely bound. The plaque color may vary from red with a small amount of scale (Figure 17), a white plaque with thick scale (Figures 18, 19 and 20), to a grayish white color (Figure 21), due to very thick adherent scale that is sometimes seen in untreated psoriasis.

A useful test to establish the diagnosis, if there is doubt, particularly when the lesion is a red non-scaly plaque, is to excoriate the lesion with a wooden spatula. If the lesion is psoriatic then the red plaque is turned into a white scaly one (Figures 22 and 23). This is due to the fact that the keratin in psoriasis is very loosely bound. If the keratin scales are lying flat, then visible light will pass through the keratin layers, and, when it reaches the dilated capillaries, the red part of the spectrum will be reflected, giving a red appearance to the plaque. However, when the loose keratin scales in psoriasis are disrupted by excoriation, the keratin lies at all angles to the surface and thus light (of all wavelengths) is reflected, giving a white appearance. A further useful sign if there is doubt about the diagnosis is to excoriate the lesion more vigorously and remove all the loosely bound keratin. A shiny surface (Figure 24) with capillary bleeding points (Figure 25 and 26) will then appear (Auspitz's sign).

Psoriasis tends to be a symmetrical eruption (Figures 27–30), and symmetry is a very helpful feature in establishing a diagnosis. Although unilateral psoriasis (Figure 31) may occur, it is the exception rather than the rule.

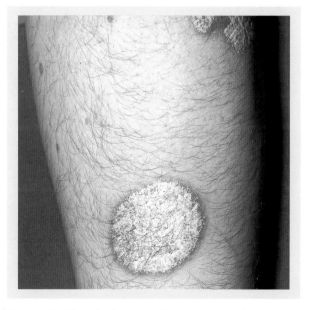

Figure 16 Sharply demarcated plaque with white scale

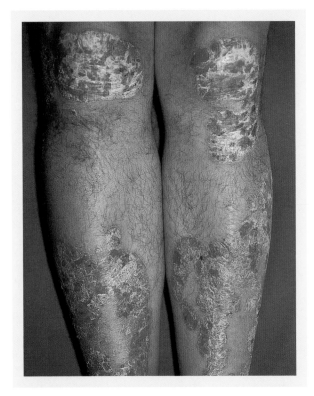

Figure 17 Symmetrical red plaques of psoriasis with minimal scaling

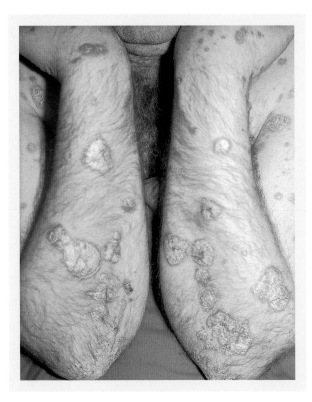

Figure 18 Thick plaques, some with white, and others with gray scale

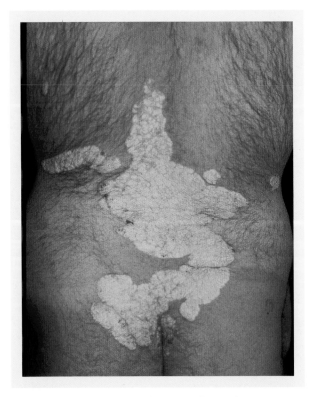

Figure 19 Thick, white adherent scale on plaques

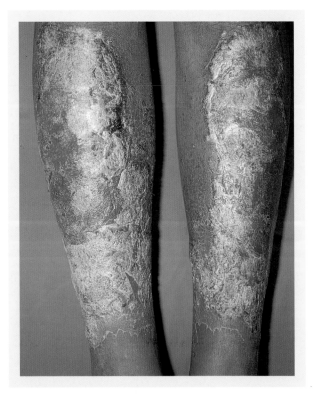

Figure 20 Symmetrical thick white/gray adherent scale in untreated psoriasis

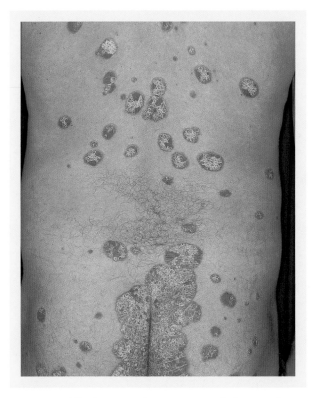

Figure 21 Thick gray scales in untreated chronic plaque psoriasis

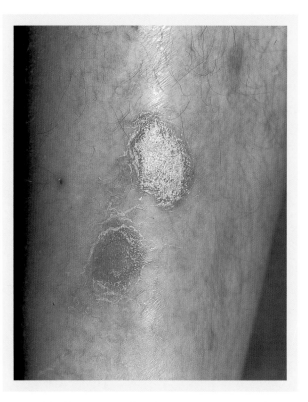

Figure 22 Excoriation of a plaque converting a red, non-scaly surface into a white, scaly one

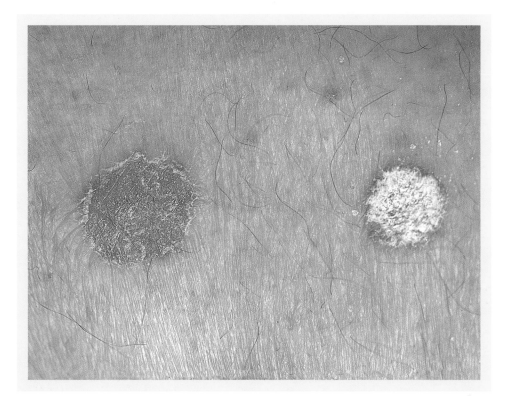

Figure 23 Two similar red plaques of psoriasis. The one on the right has been excoriated to produce a white scaly lesion

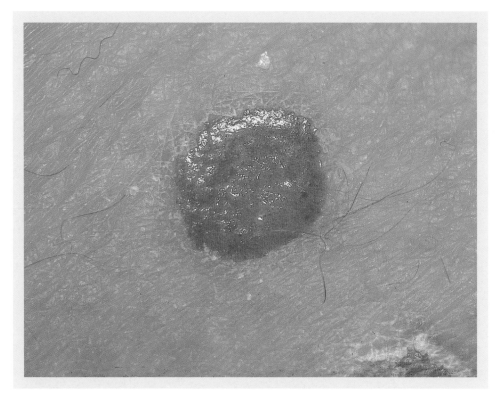

Figure 24 Glistening surface of a plaque of psoriasis after removal of scale

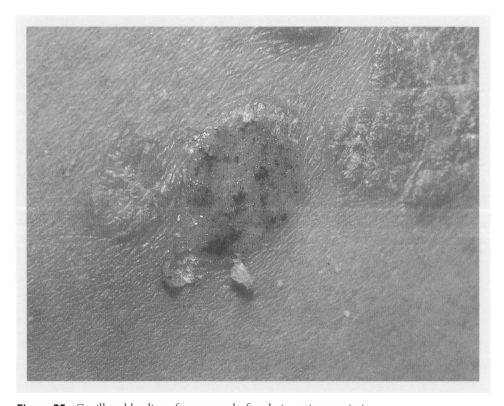

Figure 25 Capillary bleeding after removal of scale in active psoriasis

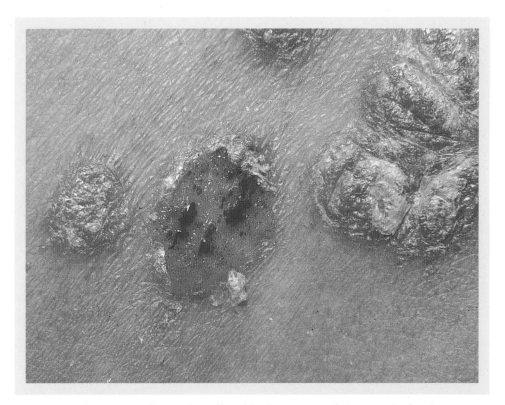

Figure 26 Glistening surface and capillary bleeding points after removal of scale in active psoriasis. Typical adjacent plaques of psoriasis

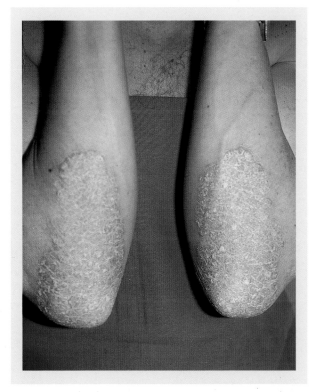

Figure 27 Symmetrical plaques on the elbows and extensor forearms

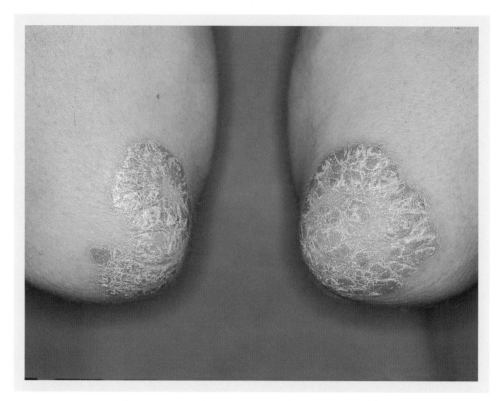

Figure 28 Symmetrical plaques on elbows at one of the commonest sites

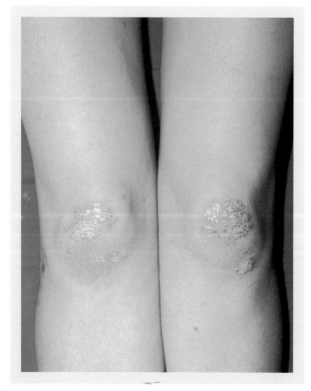

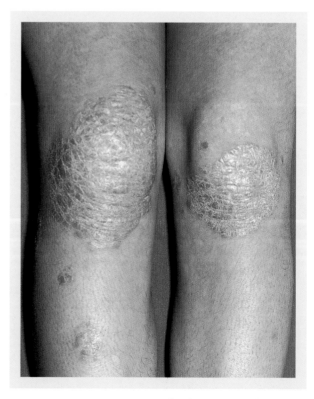

Figure 29 Symmetrical plaques on a common site, the knees

Figure 30 Large symmetrical plaques on the knees, another of the common sites

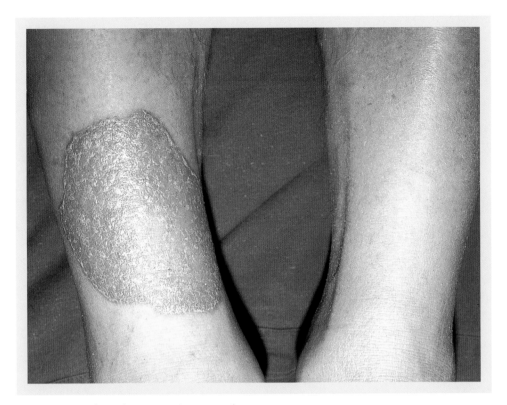

Figure 31 Unilateral psoriasis. An unusual presentation

7

Sites and clinical patterns

PLAQUE PSORIASIS

This is the commonest form of psoriasis, and is the type seen in approximately 90% of patients. Plaque psoriasis is the usual form of presentation in adults. The lesions vary in number from one to several (Figures 31–36) and in size from 0.5 to 30 cm or more (Figures 32–38). If the disease is active, the plaques will merge to form large confluent areas of psoriasis (Figures 39–43). The commonest sites for psoriasis are the extensor surfaces of the elbows (Figures 27 and 28), knees (Figures 29 and 30) and scalp, but the skin on any part of the body may be involved, either with or without lesions elsewhere. Another common site is over the sacrum (Figures 44 and 45). The face is the site least likely to be involved. The disease presents as symmetrical well-demarcated red scaly plaques (Figures 27–30).

The extent of involvement may vary from less than 1 to 100% of the skin surface (when it is termed erythrodermic psoriasis). The course of plaque psoriasis varies. It may resolve spontaneously (even after

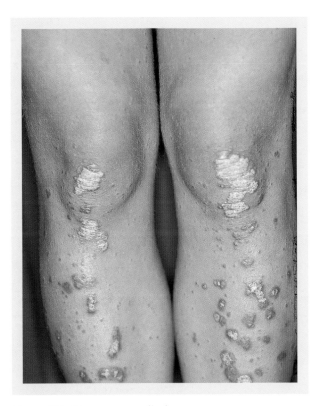

Figure 32 Numerous small plaques

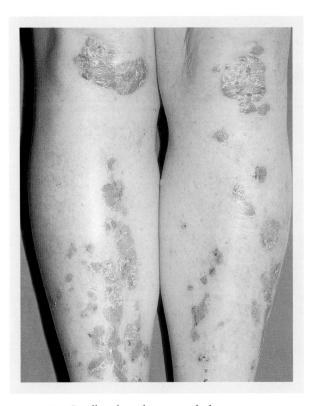

Figure 33 Small and moderate-sized plaques

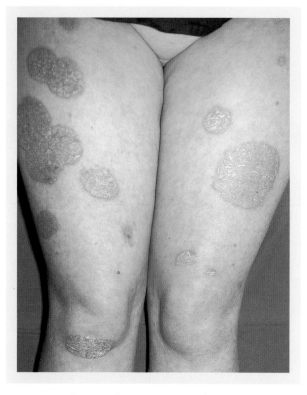

Figure 34 Plaques of various sizes with minimal scale on the thighs

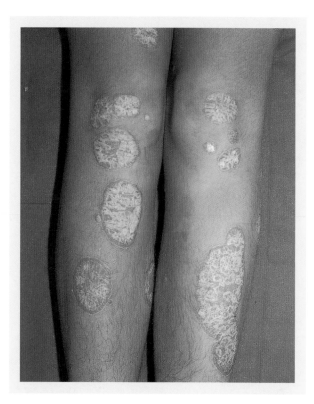

Figure 35 Various sized plaques with white scale on the legs

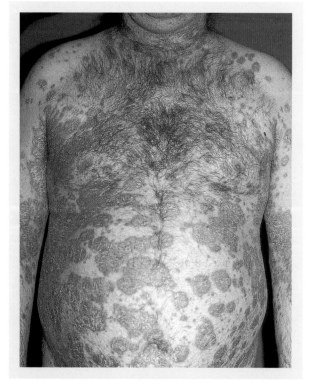

Figure 36 Extensive involvement on the trunk. Numerous large plaques

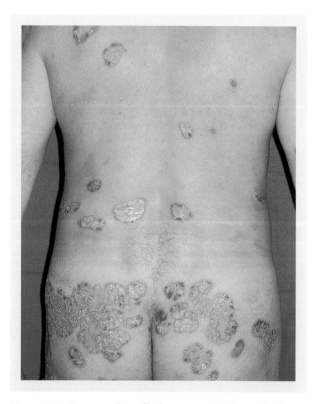

Figure 37 Large and small plaques on the lower back

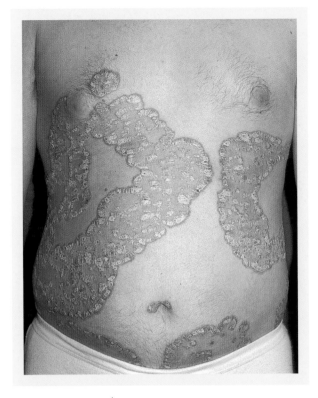

Figure 38 Large plaques

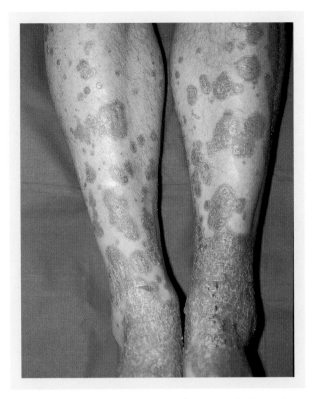

Figure 39 Plaques becoming confluent on the lower legs

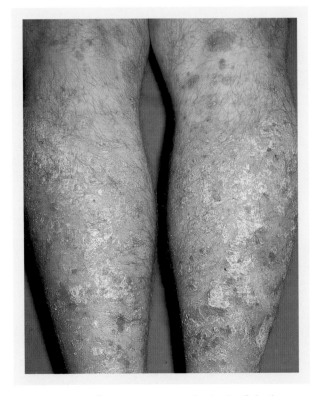

Figure 40 Confluent psoriasis on the back of the legs

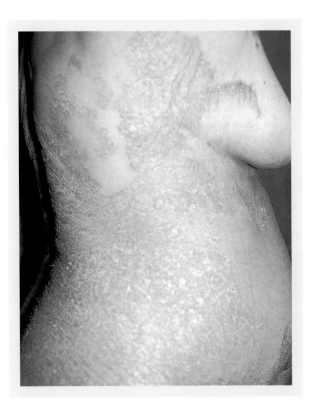

Figure 41 Extensive confluent psoriasis on the trunk

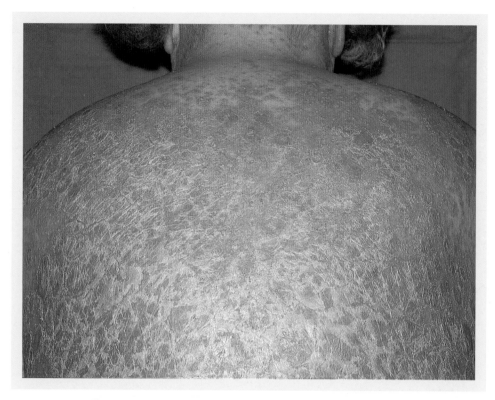

Figure 42 Confluent psoriasis on the back. Nearly all the skin is involved

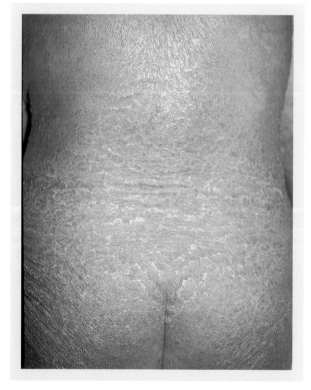

Figure 43 Confluent psoriasis – only small areas of non-involved skin are visible

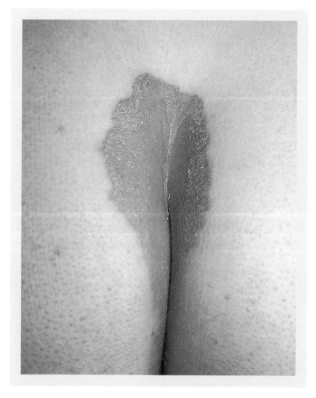

Figure 44 Psoriasis over the sacral area, another common site for psoriasis

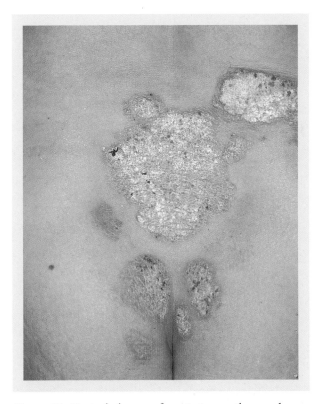

Figure 45 Typical plaques of psoriasis over the sacral area, a common site

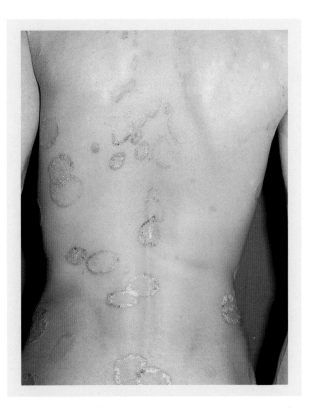

Figure 46 Resolving psoriasis, presenting as annular lesions

many years), it may remain static, or it may progress with the enlargement of existing plaques and the appearance of new ones. When plaque psoriasis clears, particularly when this occurs spontaneously, it tends to clear from the center and the situation is reached when only the periphery of the plaque remains, giving rise to annular lesions (Figure 46). The latter type of lesion, therefore, tends to imply a good prognosis.

Temporary loss of pigment is not infrequent when psoriasis clears, giving rise to white macular areas (Figures 47–49).

GUTTATE PSORIASIS

This presents with the sudden appearance of small red papules, predominantly on the trunk (Figures 50–52). New lesions may continue to appear over the next month and may involve the limbs, face and scalp. The lesions tend to persist for 2–3 months, then resolve spontaneously. Thus, guttate psoriasis tends to be a self-limiting disorder. The lesions are approximately 0.5 cm and have little scale (Figures 50–53), although, if excoriated, white silvery scale

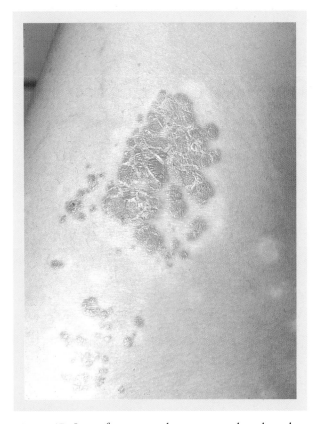

Figure 47 Loss of pigment where psoriasis has cleared

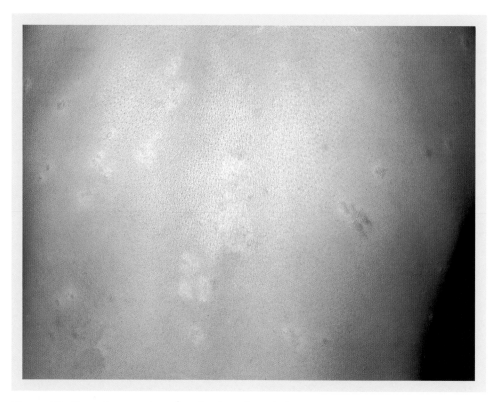

Figure 48 Hypopigmentation after clearing of psoriasis

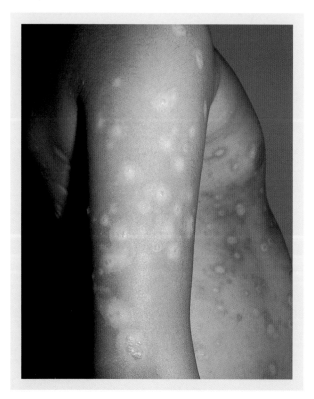

Figure 49 Hypopigmented areas at sites of previous psoriasis. These changes are more obvious in dark-skinned persons

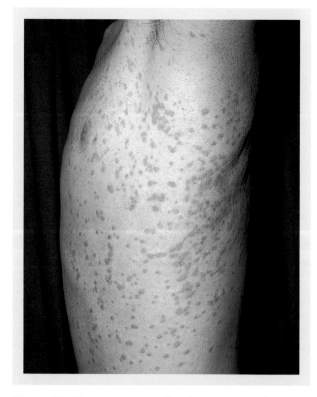

Figure 50 Guttate psoriasis. Papules on the trunk

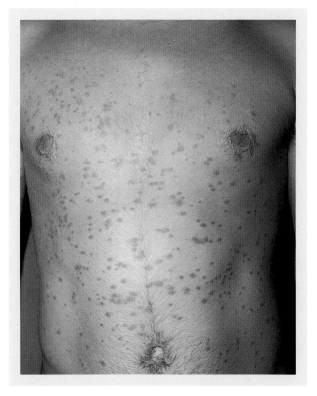

Figure 51 Guttate psoriasis on the chest and upper abdomen

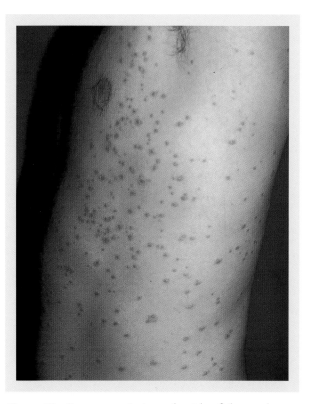

Figure 52 Guttate psoriasis on the side of the trunk

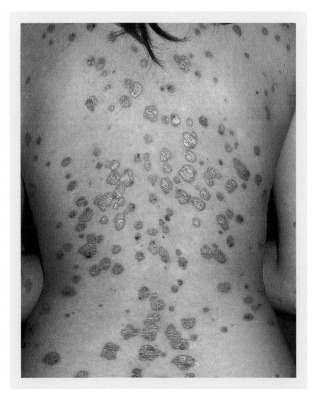

Figure 53 Guttate psoriasis on the back. Active disease with lesions showing a tendency to enlarge

will usually appear. Guttate psoriasis occurs more commonly in children, adolescents and young adults. Characteristically, it is preceded by a streptococcal sore throat. Some individuals have recurrent attacks of guttate psoriasis.

Very occasionally, guttate psoriasis lesions may enlarge (Figure 53) and persist; the disease then takes on the characteristics of chronic plaque disease (Figure 54).

CHRONIC PLAQUE COMBINED WITH GUTTATE PSORIASIS

Patients who have established chronic plaque psoriasis sometimes develop typical guttate psoriasis. The guttate psoriasis lasts the usual 3 months, and the chronic plaque lesions may remain unaltered. On other occasions, the chronic plaque lesions enlarge when guttate psoriasis appears, and the disease generally becomes more active. In this situation, the enlarged plaques may not revert to their previous state when the guttate lesions resolve.

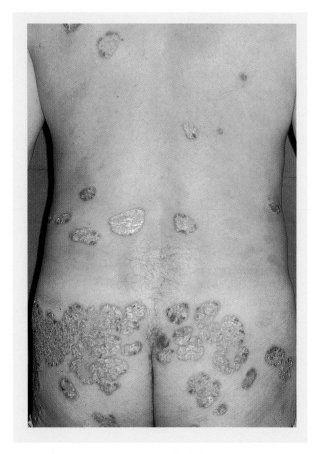

Figure 54 Guttate psoriasis which has evolved into the plaque form

KOEBNER PHENOMENON

As previously described in the section on etiology, the Koebner phenomenon is psoriasis appearing at the sites of trauma to the skin. The Koebner phenomenon does not occur in all patients. A patient may show variations in time between being Koebner-positive and Koebner-negative. The nature of the injury is not specific. The clinical appearance of psoriasis in the Koebner phenomenon follows the site of injury. It may follow friction from tight clothing (Figure 55), follow a linear scratch (Figure 56), or occur at the site of an operation (Figure 57).

ERYTHRODERMIC PSORIASIS

This term is used when all the skin is involved in the psoriatic process (Figure 58). The skin is bright red, but the scaling is different from that seen in chronic plaque. There are no thick adherent white scales; instead there is superficial scaling. In erythrodermic psoriasis, the psoriatic process is at its most active, with increased proliferation and loss of maturation of the keratinocytes, and their increased transit time; this in turn leads to abnormal keratin production, and the keratin that is formed is loosely bound and quickly shed.

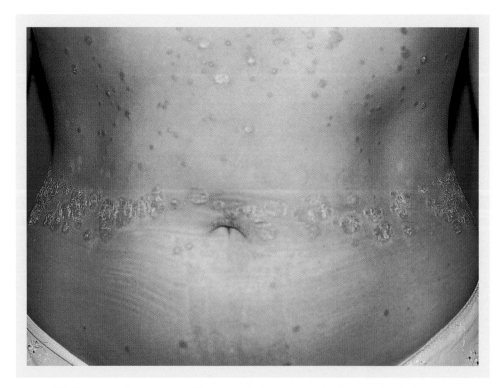

Figure 55 Koebner phenomenon. Linear psoriasis on the waist from tight clothing

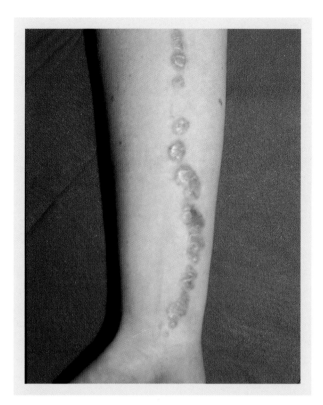

Figure 56 Koebner-positive. Linear psoriasis from a scratch

Patients with erythrodermic psoriasis lose excessive heat because of generalized vasodilatation of the cutaneous vessels. This may give rise to hypothermia. Therefore, patients with erythrodermic psoriasis are often found to be shivering, in an attempt to raise their body temperature. Edema of the limbs develops because of the vasodilatation and loss of protein from the blood vessels into the tissues. High-output cardiac failure and impaired hepatic and renal function may also occur in long-standing erythroderma.

Erythrodermic psoriasis usually develops from extensive chronic plaque or generalized pustular psoriasis, and implies that the disease is becoming more active.

Erythrodermic psoriasis is usually seen in young and middle-aged adults, but may occur at any age. There may be no exogenous trigger factors. However, known triggers include severe 'sunburn' (either from artificial ultraviolet light lamps or the sun), withdrawal of systemic steroids, irritation of the skin from coal tar and dithranol, and systemic infections. HIV infection may cause an exacerbation of existing psoriasis and this may become erythrodermic. Erythrodermic psoriasis is now seen less

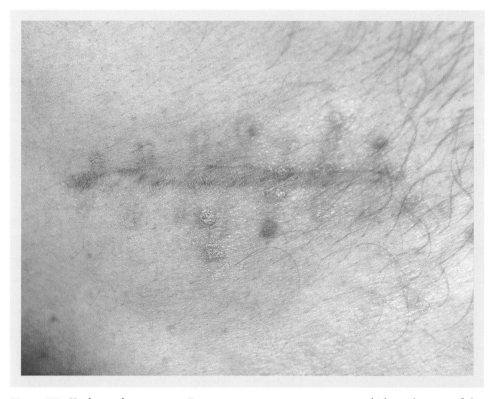

Figure 57 Koebner phenomenon. Psoriasis at an operation site, particularly at the sites of the sutures

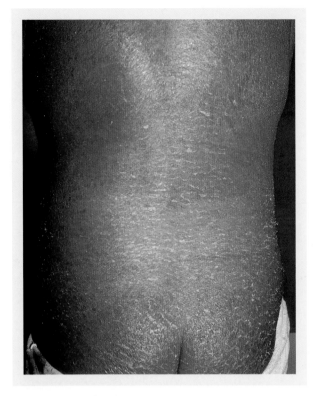

Figure 58 Erythrodermic psoriasis

commonly because treatments for extensive plaque psoriasis have improved over the last 30 years.

Erythrodermic psoriasis implies active disease and, therefore, usually a poor prognosis, particularly if there is no specific trigger. In the majority of patients, the disease reverts to extensive plaque disease with a tendency towards further bouts of erythrodermic disease. If there is a specific trigger, then the prognosis is better and, provided the trigger can be avoided, there may be no further episodes of erythroderma.

PUSTULAR PSORIASIS

There are two distinct entities to which the term pustular psoriasis refers. The first is generalized pustular psoriasis and the second is localized pustular psoriasis.

Generalized pustular psoriasis

This is an extremely rare form of psoriasis. It is usually preceded by other forms of the disease, e.g. chronic plaque, seborrheic (flexural), localized pustular psoriasis of the palms and soles, or acral

psoriasis (see below). Generalized pustular psoriasis is usually seen in middle age and the sexes are equally affected.

The triggers which may be associated with generalized pustular psoriasis include withdrawal of systemic steroids, hypocalcemia, infections (particularly those of the upper respiratory tract) and local irritants, e.g. dithranol and ultraviolet light.

Four clinical patterns of generalized pustular psoriasis have been described, but, as is usual with clinical descriptive dermatology, there is some overlap between them.

The first is still sometimes referred to as the von Zumbusch pattern after the person who first described it. It consists of a generalized eruption of sudden onset, with erythema and pustules (Figures 59–61). There is constitutional upset and a leukocytosis. The pustules are often superseded by sheets of scaling. The eruption lasts for a few weeks and then tends to revert to its previous state or it may transform into erythrodermic psoriasis (Figure 62). Subsequent episodes of generalized pustulation may follow.

An *annular* form of generalized pustular psoriasis may occur in which the pustules form in the periphery of red annular lesions. The annular form of the disease is probably a less severe form of the generalized von Zumbusch pattern, and tends to be more persistent.

An *exanthematic* form of generalized pustular psoriasis tends to occur after a viral infection and consists of widespread pustules with generalized plaque psoriasis. However, unlike the von Zumbusch pattern, there is no constitutional upset and the disorder tends not to recur.

A *localized* area of pustulation may occur in plaque psoriasis on the trunk and limbs (Figure 63) (distinct from the chronic form on the palms and soles). The localized area usually occurs after the application of an irritant, e.g. dithranol, or following the withdrawal of potent topical steroids. This localized form may simply be an extension of chronic plaque psoriasis but with an increase in the chemotactic factors for neutrophils.

At present, it is not known whether there are distinct pathogenic mechanisms in generalized pustular psoriasis, compared to chronic plaque disease, determined by genetic variation. Alternatively, the pustular phase is simply a more acute form of psoriasis with a greater release of chemotactic factors for neutrophils.

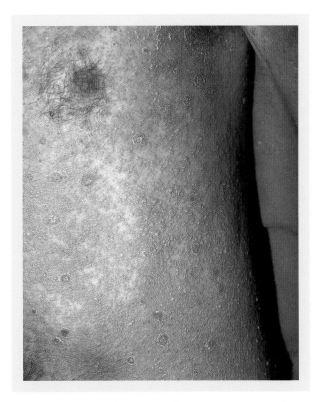

Figure 59 Generalized pustular psoriasis. Confluent erythematous areas with numerous small pustules

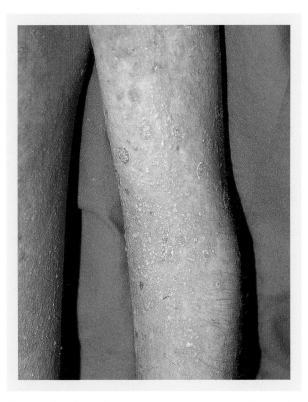

Figure 60 Generalized pustular psoriasis – small pustules and superficial erosions

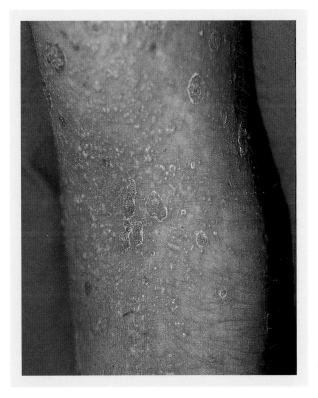

Figure 61 Numerous small pustules on erythematous background in generalized pustular psoriasis

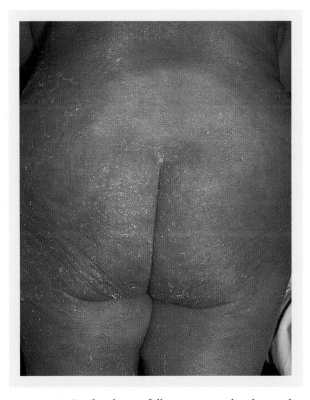

Figure 62 Erythroderma following generalized pustular psoriasis

43

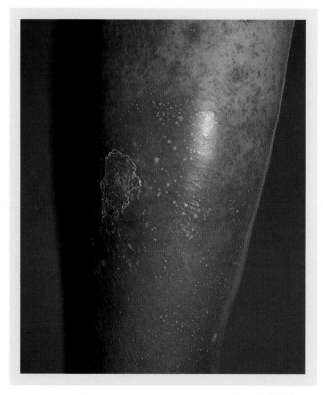

Figure 63 An area of localized pustular psoriasis on the leg

Localized pustular psoriasis

This term is used for a distinct clinical entity affecting the palms and soles (Figures 64 and 65). It is sometimes also referred to as persistent palmoplantar pustulosis. The disorder is usually seen in young and middle-aged adults and is more common in females.

The characteristic lesion is a well-defined area of redness and scaling with pustules. Frequently, reddish-brown maculopapular lesions are also present (Figures 66–68) which are resolving pustules.

The discoid lesions may be solitary or multiple. They may remain the same size or occasionally enlarge and may coalesce and affect large areas of the palms and soles. Sometimes there is no definite edge to the affected area, and it is mainly a collection of pustules with associated scaling and erythema.

Localized pustular psoriasis may affect both palms and soles (in the same individual) or only the palms or soles. It is usually bilateral and symmetrical (Figure 65), but unilateral presentation may also occur. It is a very persistent condition; the lesions cleared in only one-third of patients in a 10-year follow-up study.

The relationship of localized pustular psoriasis to other forms of psoriasis is still unsettled. In favor of the localized palmar/plantar lesions being a form of psoriasis is the higher incidence of plaque psoriasis in patients with localized pustular psoriasis, compared to a control population. However, there is no reported increase of the HLA antigens, B13, B17, CW6 and DR7 in localized pustular psoriasis. There is also no increase in DNA-synthesizing cells in the epidermis of the uninvolved skin, as occurs in the uninvolved skin of patients with plaque psoriasis.

ACRAL PSORIASIS

This variant of psoriasis begins on the fingers (Figure 69), and less frequently the toes (Figures 70 and 71), around the nails as small red scaly plaques. Pustules may be seen and there is associated nail dystrophy. Underlying bone changes may occur in the chronic form of the disease. Proximal progression of the psoriasis tends to occur, and plaque lesions may develop at distinct sites. Eventual progression into generalized pustular psoriasis may follow.

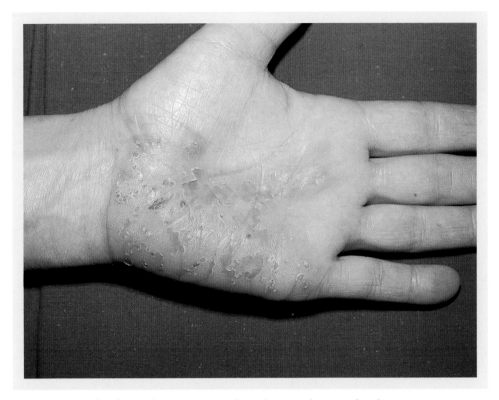

Figure 64 Localized pustular psoriasis on the palm – erythema and scaling

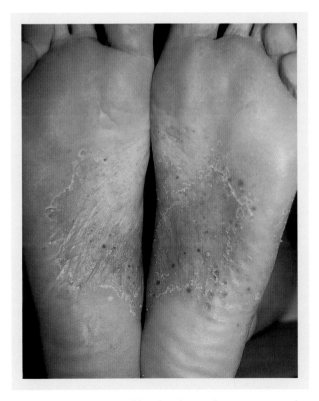

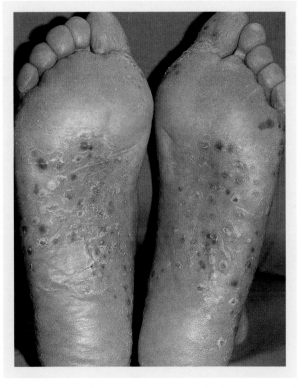

Figure 65 Symmetrical localized pustular psoriasis on the soles

Figure 66 Pustules and 'brown papules', characteristic of localized pustular psoriasis on the soles

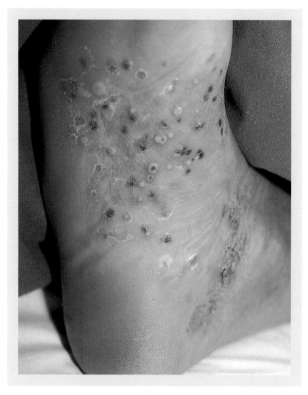

Figure 67   Severe pustulation in localized pustular psoriasis

SEBORRHEIC PSORIASIS

In this form of psoriasis, the lesions tend to occur at the same sites as seborrheic eczema, i.e. nose, medial cheeks, nasolabial folds, eyebrows, forehead and chin (Figures 72 and 73) intertrigenous areas (Figures 74–76) and the center of the chest. If there are no lesions elsewhere, then it may be difficult to distinguish this form of psoriasis from seborrheic eczema.

CHILDHOOD PSORIASIS

Chronic plaque psoriasis is rare in children, and guttate psoriasis is also not usually seen under the age of 5 years. One of the commonest forms of presentation in children is involvement of the genitalia (Figure 77) and perianal skin (Figure 78). This form of psoriasis tends to be persistent. Eventually, plaques of psoriasis tend to appear elsewhere on the trunk and limbs. Another form of presentation in children is of lesions appearing around the nails with an associated nail dystrophy (Figure 79). Psoriasis confined to the scalp may occur in children.

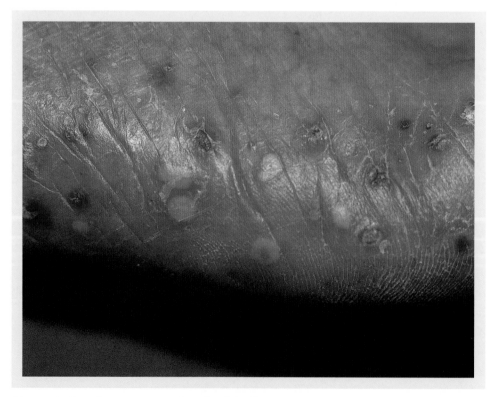

Figure 68   Pustular psoriasis on the side of the foot

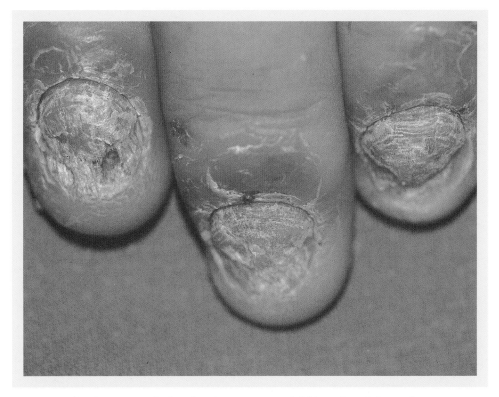

Figure 69 Acral psoriasis. Red and scaly posterior nail folds with nail dystrophy

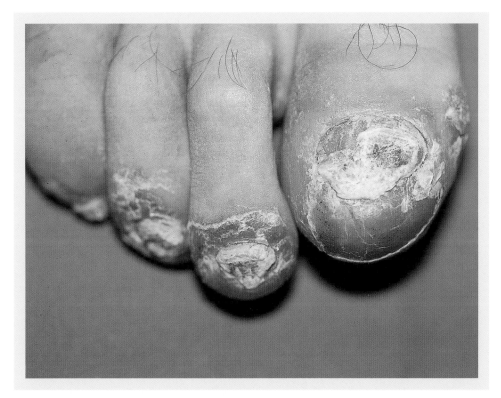

Figure 70 Acral psoriasis. Severe nail dystrophy and involvement of the nail folds

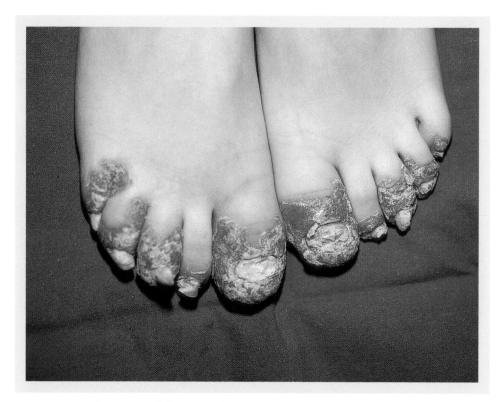

Figure 71 Acral psoriasis of the toes with nail dystrophy

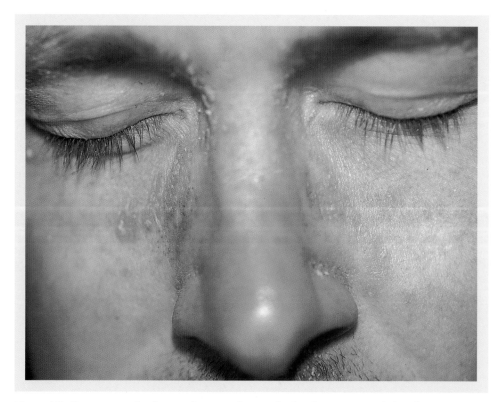

Figure 72 Psoriasis on the face at the typical sites of seborrheic eczema (seborrheic psoriasis)

DIAPER 'PSORIASIS'

This term is a misnomer as it implies that infants with this rash have psoriasis, and this is certainly not proven. The eruption usually begins between the ages of 3 and 6 months and first appears in the diaper (napkin) area (although 'cradle cap' is usually present). The rash is a confluent red area confined to the diaper area (Figure 80). A few days later small red papules appear on the trunk (Figure 80) and may also involve the limbs. These papules have the typical white scales of psoriasis. The face may be involved with red scaly areas. Unlike psoriasis, the prognosis for this eruption in infancy is good and the rash responds well to treatment and tends to disappear after the age of 1 year.

Some reports have claimed that, although the rash in infancy disappears, it is a form of psoriasis and that there is a higher incidence of psoriasis in later life. However, this has been disputed in other reports. In addition, one study has shown that incidence of HLA antigens B13, B17 and B37 is no higher in infants with diaper 'psoriasis' compared to normal individuals. The word psoriasis should

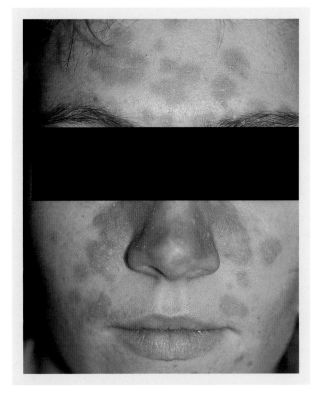

Figure 73 Seborrheic psoriasis on the face

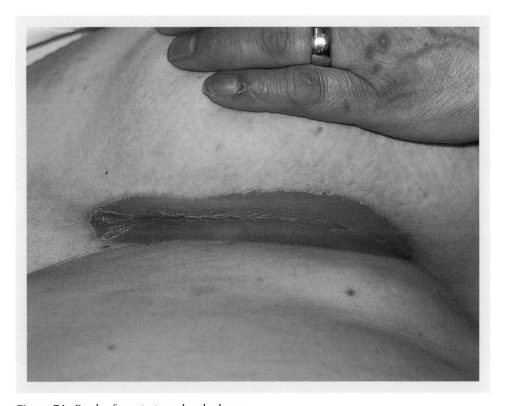

Figure 74 Patch of psoriasis under the breast

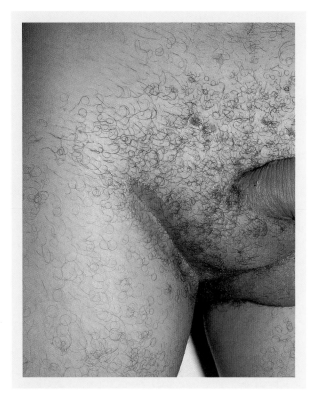

Figure 75 Psoriasis localized to the intertriginous area of the groin

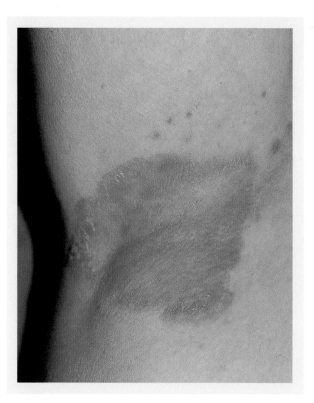

Figure 76 Discrete patch of psoriasis in the axilla

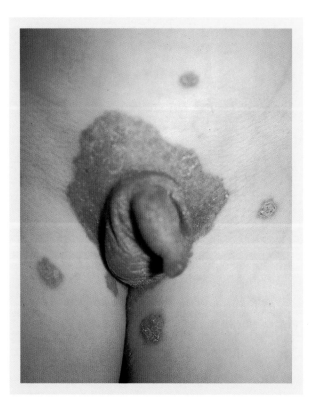

Figure 77 Psoriasis of the genitalia and pubic area, common sites in children

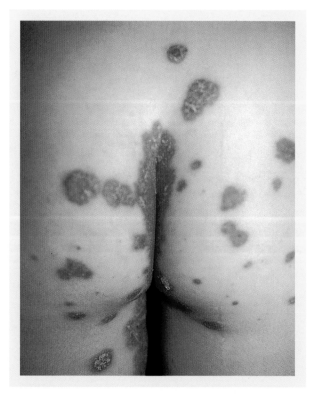

Figure 78 Psoriasis of the natal cleft (a common site in children), with surrounding plaques

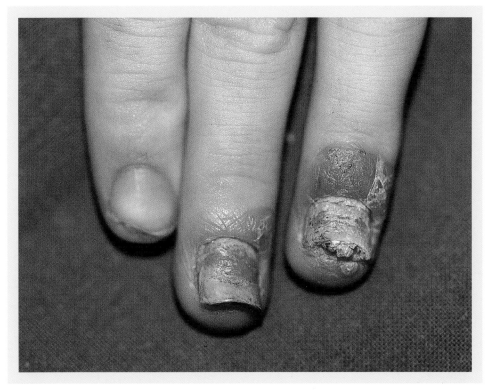

Figure 79 Acral psoriasis with nail involvement, a not uncommon presentation in childhood

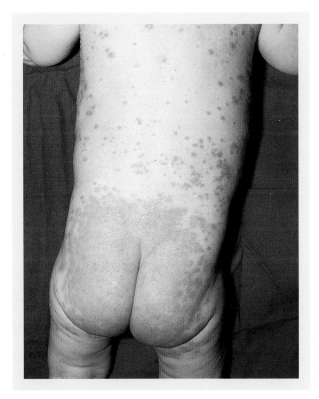

Figure 80 Confluent involvement in diaper (napkin) area, and papules and plaques on the trunk in diaper 'psoriasis'

therefore not be used for this type of eruption; a more appropriate term is seborrheic eczema of infancy.

LINEAR PSORIASIS

This is a rare form of presentation. The psoriatic lesion presents as a straight line on limbs (Figure 81), or may be limited to a dermatome on the trunk. In adults, the etiology of this form of the disease is unknown. In children it has been postulated as being due to an underlying nevus, which may predispose to the psoriatic process in susceptible individuals.

PSORIASIS AT SPECIFIC SITES

Scalp

The scalp is one of the commonest sites to develop psoriasis, and there may be no lesions elsewhere. Psoriasis of the scalp characteristically extends only to or just beyond the hair line (Figures 82 and 83). The commonest site of involvement of the scalp is behind the ears (Figures 83 and 84). Psoriasis of the

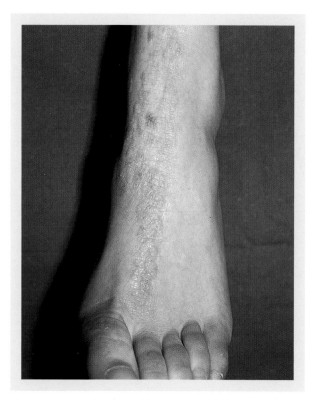

Figure 81 Linear psoriasis

scalp may present as discrete red raised scaly plaques, as found elsewhere on the trunk and limbs, or it may show diffuse scaling, or may present as very thick plaques of keratin with the scales growing along the hair shafts (Figure 85).

Hair loss with psoriasis of the scalp (Figure 86) is the exception rather than the rule. It does, however, occur with severe psoriasis, particularly the erythrodermic form of the disease. The alopecia presents as a diffuse thinning of the hair in the most severely affected areas, and may occur all over the scalp in erythrodermic psoriasis. The hair loss is reversible when the psoriasis clears, either with treatment or spontaneously.

Beard and pubic area

In patients with beards and in the pubic area (Figure 87), psoriasis may also be limited to the areas with hair. If the beard is shaved off, the psoriasis clears. No satisfactory explanation for this observation has been given.

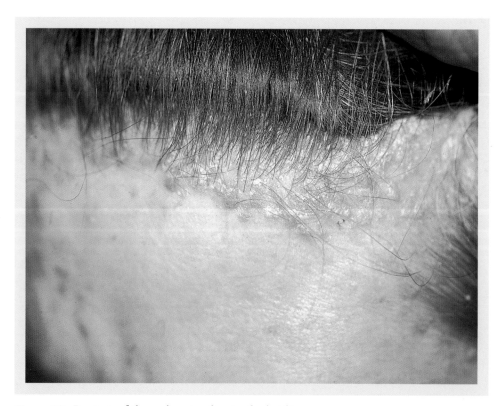

Figure 82 Psoriasis of the scalp extending to the hairline

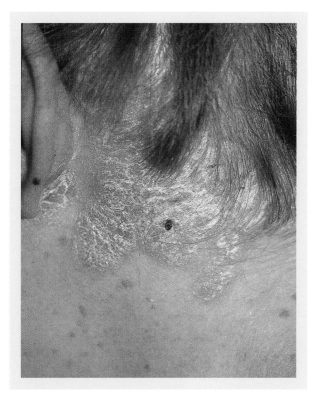

Figure 83 Extension of psoriasis just beyond the hairline in active disease

Palms and soles

The palms and soles may be involved in plaque or guttate psoriasis. Occasionally, psoriasis (distinct from localized pustular psoriasis) may only affect the palms and/or soles. The appearance of psoriasis on the palms and soles tends to be different from the lesions elsewhere and this may give rise to diagnostic difficulty. The different clinical presentation is probably due to the different structure of the skin on the palms and soles. On the occasions when guttate psoriasis affects the palms and soles, it presents as hard reddish brown papules (Figure 88). There may or may not be some scale, but, if present, it is fairly adherent, unlike the lesions elsewhere on the trunk and limbs.

Plaque psoriasis may occur on the palms and soles with or without plaque lesions elsewhere. The palms and soles may have discrete lesions (Figure 89) or there may be confluent involvement affecting all the plantar and palmar skin, including the digits (Figure 90). In the latter presentation, there is a sharp line of demarcation between the palmar and plantar involvement and the surrounding skin (Figure 91).

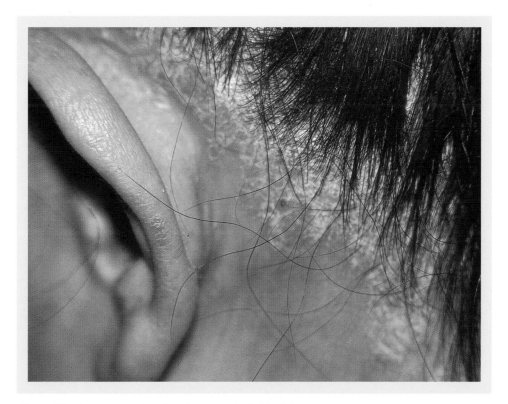

Figure 84 A common site of scalp psoriasis, behind the ear

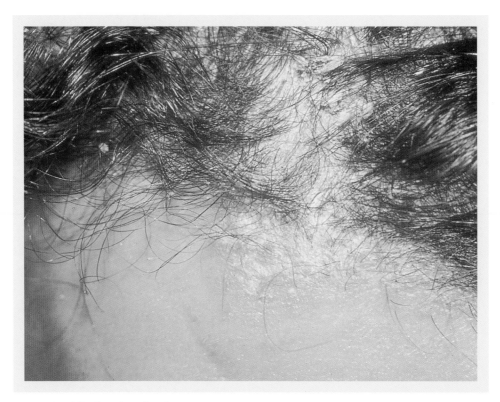

Figure 85 Thick scales of scalp psoriasis

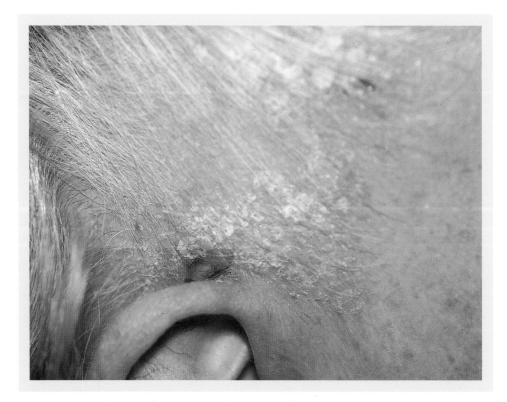

Figure 86 Hair loss in scalp psoriasis, an uncommon feature

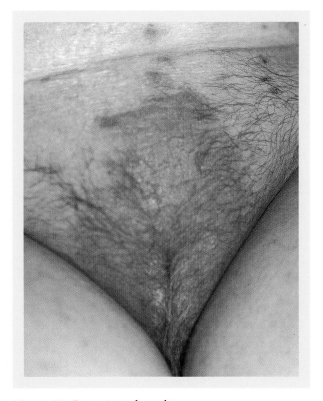

Figure 87 Psoriasis in the pubic area

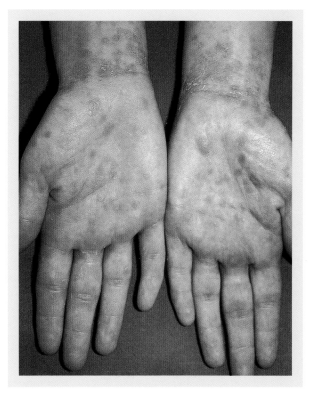

Figure 88 Guttate psoriasis on the palms

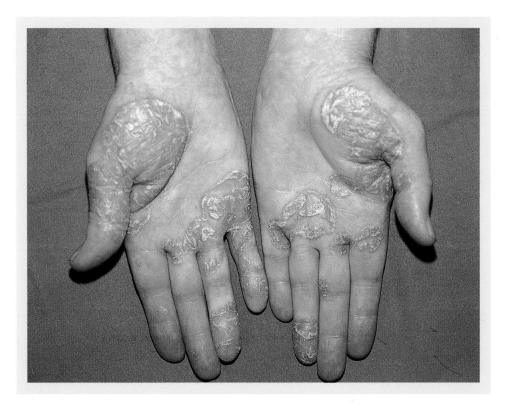

Figure 89 Localized symmetrical lesions of psoriasis on the palms. The scaling is different from plaque psoriasis elsewhere on the trunk and limbs

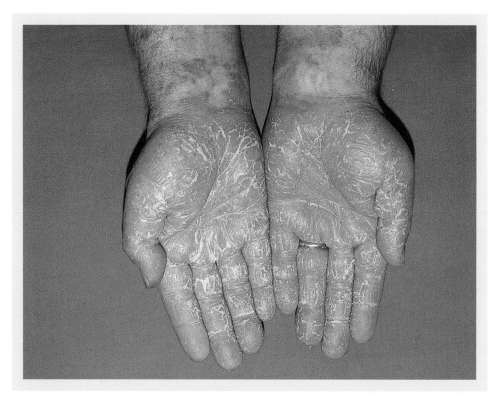

Figure 90 Confluent psoriasis on the palms

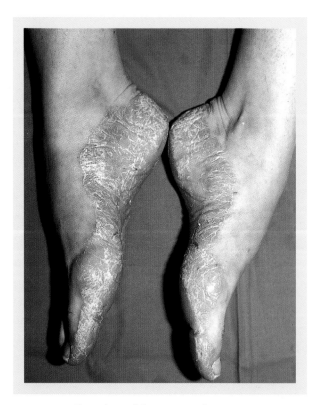

Figure 91 Sharp line of demarcation between psoriasis on the sole and the surrounding skin

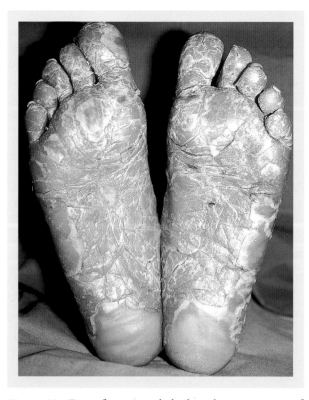

Figure 92 Deep fissures and thick scales in psoriasis of the soles

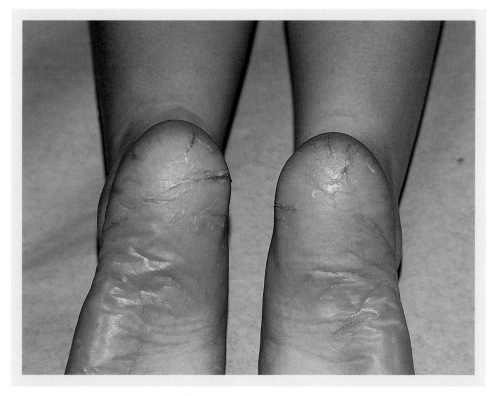

Figure 93 Fissuring in psoriasis of the soles

Another form of palmar/plantar psoriasis presents as red fissured skin (Figures 92 and 93). There may be severe limitation of movement of the hand and/or foot with this type of lesion. The typical white flaky surface characteristic of psoriasis elsewhere may be absent (Figure 93). Occasionally, psoriasis on the palms and soles may present as so-called keratoderma. In this form there is very thick gray-white keratin. Fissuring is common and painful. Involvement of the soles leads to difficulty in walking, and on the palms there is severe limitation of normal function, so everyday tasks are difficult to perform, and manual occupations are difficult to follow.

Flexures and intertriginous areas

As mentioned above, psoriasis may predominantly involve the intertriginous areas in so-called 'seborrheic psoriasis'. At other times, involvement of those sites may occur in plaque psoriasis (Figure 94). Psoriasis in an intertriginous area is often limited to the area where the folds of skin are in actual contact; there is a sharp line of demarcation between the involved and uninvolved skin (Figures 74, 75 and 76). The psoriatic lesion may be raised or flat. The skin is red and has a shiny appearance and there is

little or no scaling (Figures 74, 75, 94 and 95). This lack of scaling is due to the sweat in the intertriginous area hydrating the keratin which inhibits scaling. If the opposing skin surfaces are kept apart for any length of time, superficial scaling will appear. In intertriginous psoriasis, painful fissures may appear at the apex of the fold (Figures 95 and 96), particularly the posterior natal cleft (Figure 96). The areas involved in intertriginous psoriasis are the natal cleft, groins, axillae, submammary area, abdominal folds (in obese subjects) (Figure 95) and between the small toes.

Genitalia

The male genitalia are not an infrequent site for psoriasis. It has been reported that between 2 and 5% of male patients have psoriasis on the penis. Sometimes psoriasis only affects the penis and the correct diagnosis is often missed. The commonest site of involvement is the proximal part of the glans (Figure 97). Small red well-demarcated plaques, varying from 0.5 to 2 cm, are the typical lesions. The thick white scaling of ordinary plaque psoriasis is not usually present. In circumcized individuals, some superficial scaling may be seen, but in the uncircumcized the patches have a shiny appearance (Figure

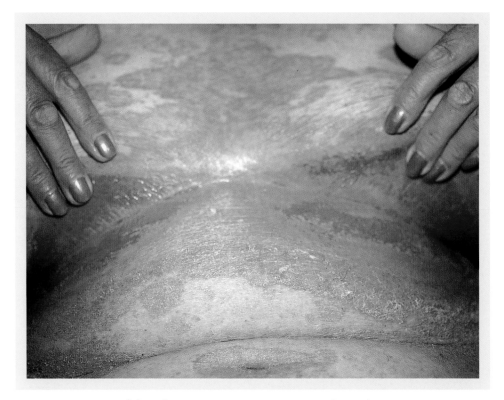

Figure 94 Psoriasis of the infra-mammary areas in extensive plaque disease

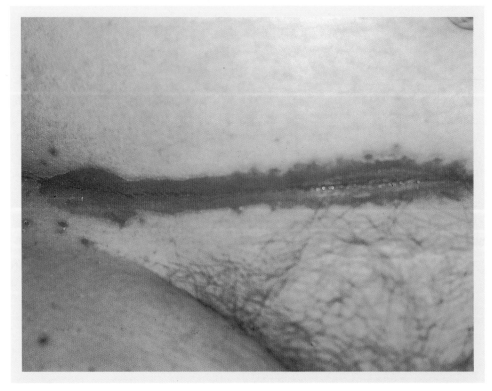

Figure 95 Psoriasis confined to the intertriginous area of an abdominal fold. Fissuring is present

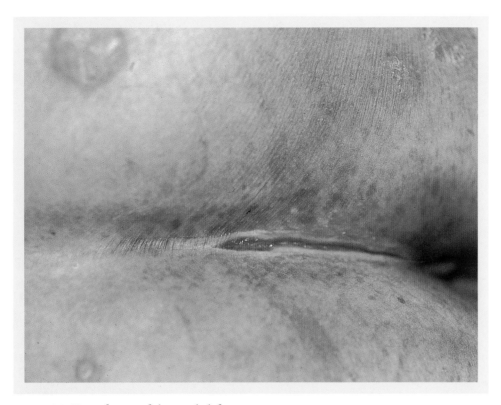

Figure 96 Deep fissure of the natal cleft

98). Plaques may also occur on the foreskin and shaft, but again thick white scales are not seen, and the appearance is that of a red patch with mild superficial scaling. Plaques and even confluent psoriasis may be present on the scrotum.

Involvement of the female genitalia also occurs. The perivulval skin may be involved with confluent red well-demarcated lesions. There is only minimal scaling (Figure 99).

Mucous membranes

Involvement of the mucous membranes in psoriasis is very rare. Scaling of the lips is sometimes seen in the erythrodermic form. Involvement of the oral cavity in generalized pustular psoriasis occurs in a small percentage of these patients. There are discrete denuded areas with white slightly elevated edges. The appearances are similar to the geographical tongue, but in psoriasis the lesions are not confined to the dorsal surface of the tongue; they may also be seen on the buccal mucosae, ventral tongue and gingivae. The histology of the oral lesions is not that of psoriasis of the skin, and the pathogenesis is likely to be different.

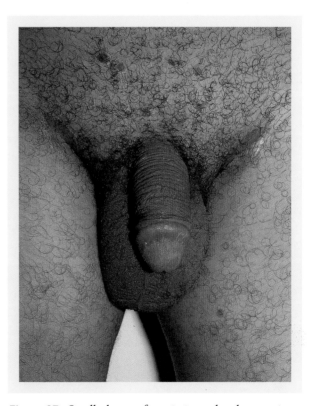

Figure 97 Small plaque of psoriasis on the glans penis

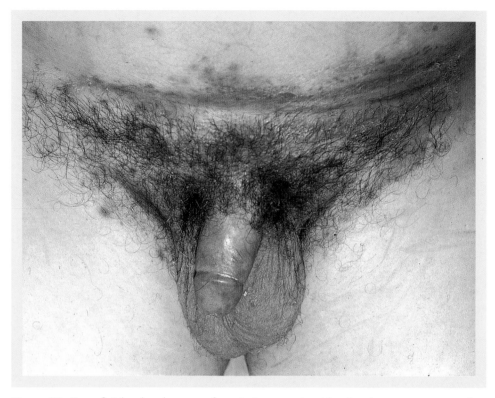

Figure 98 Superficial red scaly areas of psoriasis on penis with seborrheic psoriasis in pubic area, abdominal fold and groins

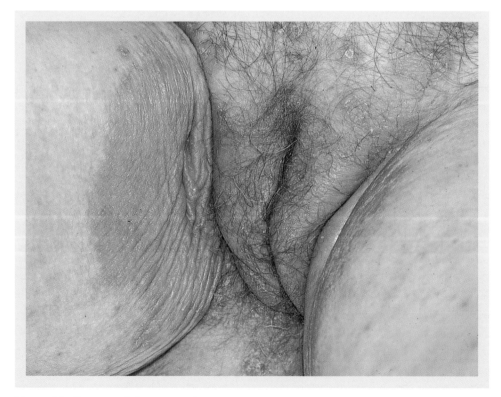

Figure 99 Psoriasis of the outer vulva

Ocular lesions are rare in psoriasis, but blepharitis and keratitis have been reported; whether these are of a primary nature, or secondary to involvement of the skin of the eyelids, is debatable.

Nails

Nail involvement in psoriasis is common. The incidence varies from 25 to 50% in reported studies. Involvement is more common in older individuals, in extensive disease and in patients with psoriatic arthropathy. The lesions may be seen in the nail plate, owing to involvement of the nail matrix, or the nail bed.

Nail pits These are one of the commonest features of psoriasis and occur more frequently in the finger than the toe nails. Pits in the nail plate are approximately the size of a pinhead and may be solitary or multiple (Figures 100 and 101). They are thought to be due to small areas of psoriatic involvement in the nail matrix.

Terminal onycholysis This is probably the second commonest feature of nail involvement and is usually seen in the finger and big toe nails. It is due to separation of the terminal nail plate from the nail bed. It presents as a whitish opaque area (Figures 101–103). Onycholysis may affect a solitary nail (Figure 102), a few, or all the nails (Figure 103). If several nails are affected, the involvement may be symmetrical. Onycholysis may only involve a small area under the nail or extend to 90% of the nail plate. If extensive, the nail may be lost, but another will regrow, and is also likely to show onycholysis.

Occasionally in onycholysis, bacteria grow under the nail plate and give rise to green (Figure 104) or black nails.

Oildrops These are brownish translucent areas seen under the nail plate (Figure 105). They are due to small areas of psoriasis, giving rise to parakeratosis of the nail bed.

Subungual hyperkeratosis This is most commonly seen in the toe nails (Figures 106 and 107). It is due to psoriasis of the nail bed with excessive production of keratin building up under the nail plate (Figure 106). It often leads to gross deformity of the nail, and destruction of the actual nail plate (Figures 107 and 108), This deformity may interfere with normal function of the fingers.

Thinning of the nail plate This is due to total involvement of the nail matrix, resulting in a thin atrophic nail plate.

Nail hemorrhages Small subungual, sometimes 'splinter', hemorrhages may be seen. These are due to trauma to the enlarged capillaries when psoriasis of the nail bed is present.

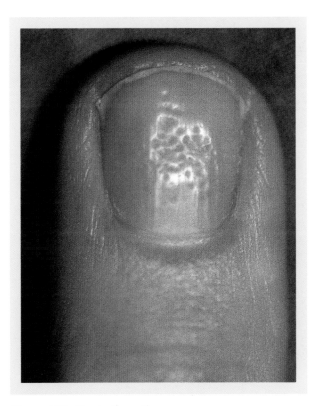

Figure 100 Pits in the nail

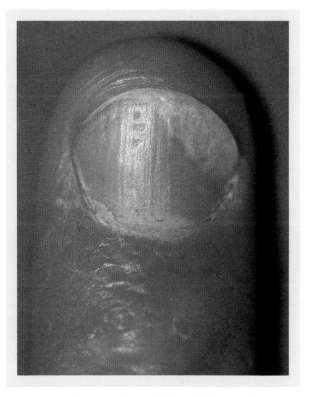

Figure 101 Pitting and onycholysis of the nail plate

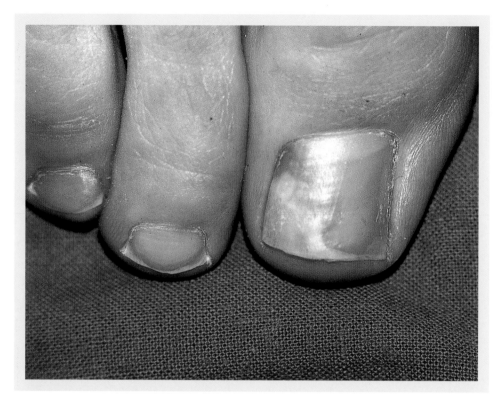

Figure 102   Onycholysis of one big toenail

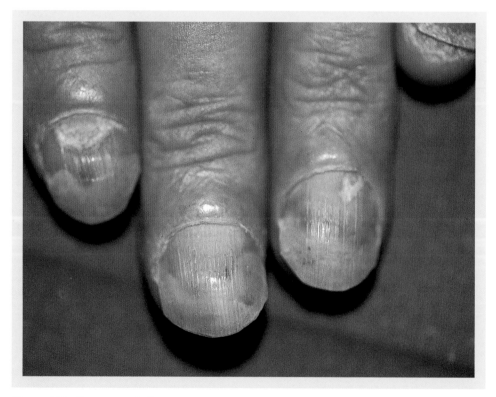

Figure 103   Severe onycholysis

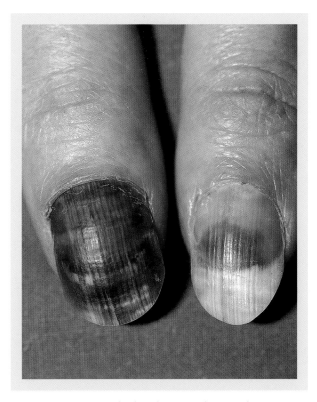

Figure 104 Greenish discoloration due to chromogenic bacteria under the nail in onycholysis

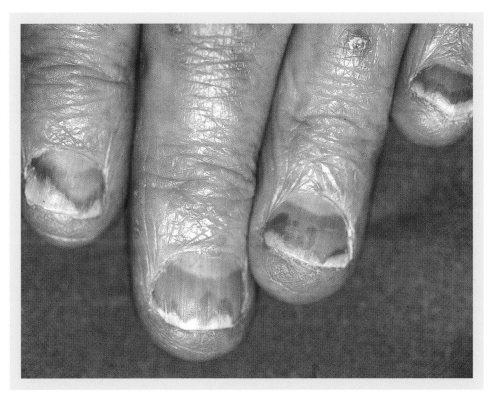

Figure 105 'Oil drop' appearance due to psoriasis of the nail bed

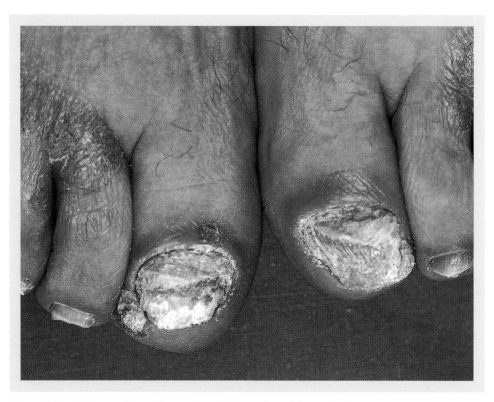

Figure 106 Subungual hyperkeratosis and dystrophy of the nail plate

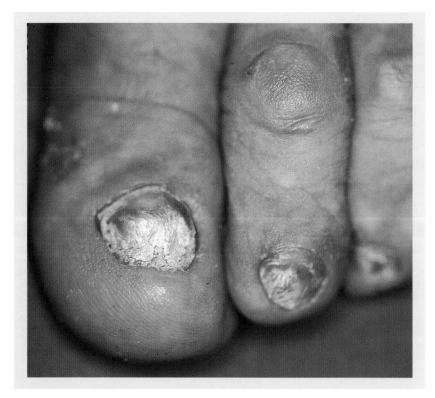

Figure 107 Severe subungual hyperkeratosis

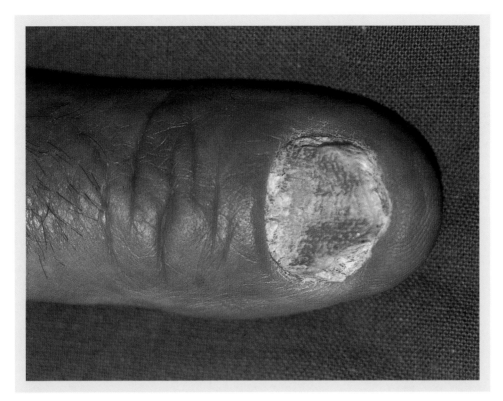

Figure 108 Dystrophy of the nail plate of the thumb with some subungual hyperkeratosis

8

Differential diagnosis

The differential diagnosis will depend on the type of psoriasis and the site involved.

CHRONIC PLAQUE PSORIASIS

Discoid eczema on the limbs in young adults presents as symmetrical discoid lesions, but in eczema there is not such a sharply defined edge between the involved and uninvolved skin. The surface of the lesion in eczema is less scaly and may be crusted.

Cutaneous T cell lymphoma (mycosis fungoides) may present as red discoid scaly lesions. However, in lymphoma the lesions are often asymmetrical, and the scaling is usually less. If there is a possibility of a lymphoma, a biopsy must be performed.

Bowen's disease usually presents as a red scaly plaque on the lower leg and occasionally mimics a solitary plaque of psoriasis. The scale in Bowen's disease is usually less than in psoriasis. A biopsy is necessary if there is doubt as to the correct diagnosis.

Pityriasis rubra pilaris is a rare disorder which presents with widespread red scaly plaques that may become confluent. Like psoriasis, there is a well-demarcated edge between involved and uninvolved skin. The disorder may be distinguished from psoriasis by the involvement of hair follicles. In pityriasis rubra pilaris, the follicles on the back of the fingers are frequently involved, giving rise to small red papules.

GUTTATE PSORIASIS

Pityriasis rosea affects a similar age group (i.e. 10–30 years), and also occurs predominantly on the trunk. However, in pityriasis rosea the lesions are usually oval and have centripetal scaling. However, occasionally in pityriasis rosea the lesions are predominantly papular, and the diagnosis may then depend on the history and presence of a herald patch, and the type of scaling.

Secondary syphilis in its papular form is another eruption of sudden onset seen in young adults. However, in syphilis involvement of the palms, soles and face is common. If there is any doubt, serology tests for syphilis must be performed.

Occasionally *endogenous eczema* (particularly the seborrheic variety) may present as small red scaly papules and patches on the trunk. An eczematous eruption is usually less papular, but white silvery scales may be present in seborrheic eczema lesions.

The chronic form of *pityriasis lichenoides* presents as small red scaly papules. The distribution of pityriasis lichenoides differs from that of guttate psoriasis in that it is not predominantly on the trunk. The type of scale on the surface of the lesion is also different in pityriasis lichenoides, as it is more adherent.

ERYTHRODERMIC PSORIASIS

Eczema and a *cutaneous T cell lymphoma* may also present as erythroderma. The appearance may be the same whatever the disease. A preceding history of eczema or psoriasis will be helpful in establishing the correct diagnosis, otherwise a biopsy will be necessary, particularly to diagnose the lymphoma.

GENERALIZED PUSTULAR PSORIASIS

Subcorneal pustular dermatosis, if widespread, may have to be considered in the differential diagnosis, but in this disorder the pustules are often relatively large (e.g. 1 cm) and do not have the associated redness and scaling. Constitutional upset is not a feature of subcorneal pustular dermatosis.

Pemphigus foliaceus may have pustular lesions and be very extensive. The areas of involvement may also be red, scaly and slightly exudative.

Impetigo, if generalized, presents with widespread pustules, erythema and crusting. Swabs for bacteriology and biopsy will establish the diagnosis.

Migratory necrolytic erythema is a very rare disorder which may be generalized and have serpiginous lesions. The tongue is red and sore and the involvement is confluent, unlike the patchy lesions in psoriasis. Migratory necrolytic erythema is usually associated with a glucagonoma and so diabetes is usually present.

Widespread *candidal* infection in immunosuppressed patients may also present with widespread erythema and pustulation.

LOCALIZED PUSTULAR PSORIASIS

Infected eczema on the palms and soles may have a similar appearance to localized pustular psoriasis. Bacteriological tests may be needed to distinguish between the two conditions.

Fungal infection on the soles may be localized and produce vesicles and pustules. Therefore, specimens for mycology should always be taken if either condition is suspected.

ACRAL PSORIASIS

Herpes simplex, *streptococcal* and *candidal* infections have to be considered in the early stages when only one finger may be involved. The appropriate pathology tests should establish the diagnosis. Periungual eczema may also give a similar picture, but pustulation is unlikely unless secondary infection is present.

SEBORRHEIC PSORIASIS

Seborrheic eczema is the obvious differential diagnosis. It may be extremely difficult to distinguish between the two conditions unless there are typical lesions of psoriasis elsewhere (including nail involvement). As has been mentioned in the introduction, the nosology of seborrheic eczema and its relationship to psoriasis may need to be redefined. It is possi-

ble that the features of so-called seborrheic eczema are simply a variant of psoriasis. It is illogical to call the condition 'psoriasis', if the more classical features of the disease are present elsewhere, and 'eczema', if these other features are absent. It is likely that in the future, as the pathogenesis and genotypes, in relation to phenotypes, are better understood, the nosology of this type of eruption will be established rather than relying solely on clinical features.

CHILDHOOD PSORIASIS

As involvement of the genitalia, groins and perianal skin are common sites for psoriasis in children, the most likely differential diagnosis includes *seborrheic eczema* and *candidal infection*. Seborrheic eczema is uncommon in children (over the age of 2 years); lesions of psoriasis elsewhere and nail involvement help to establish the diagnosis. If there is involvement of the nails, then candidal and dermatophyte infections must be excluded by mycology tests.

SCALP PSORIASIS

Seborrheic eczema is the commonest disorder to mimic psoriasis of the scalp. If there are no lesions elsewhere, it may be impossible to distinguish between the two conditions. Psoriasis tends to give thicker lesions with more scale, and the lesions are more discrete, but these are not absolute distinguishing features. If hair loss is present *fungal infections* (particularly in children) will have to be excluded.

As a general rule, psoriatic hair loss does not give rise to scarring and thus can be distinguished from *discoid lupus erythematosus*.

PSORIASIS OF THE PALMS AND SOLES

Both the discrete discoid lesions, and the confluent involvement, of the palms and soles have to be distinguished from *chronic endogenous eczema*. In addition, both eczema and psoriasis may give rise to keratoderma (thick hyperkeratotic lesions) on the palms and soles. In confluent forms of psoriasis, there is a sharper line of demarcation between the involved and uninvolved skin compared to eczema. If the blisters are present or there is a history of vesiculation, this favors eczema.

Reiter's disease, which consists of urethritis, arthritis, ocular, skin and oral lesions, commonly presents with hyperkeratotic plaques on the palms and soles. The presence or history of urethritis, ocular and oral lesions should help to distinguish between psoriasis and Reiter's disease.

FLEXURAL PSORIASIS

Seborrheic eczema (as discussed above, under seborrheic psoriasis) is the commonest disorder to be distinguished from psoriasis in intertriginous areas.

Fungal infections and *erythrasma* may also be confined to flexural or intertriginous areas. Erythrasma presents as sharply demarcated lesions in the groins and axillae, tends to have a reddish brown color and fluoresces coral pink with ultraviolet light. Fungal infections in the axillae and submammary region are relatively rare, but common in the groins. The lesions tend to have a raised red scaly edge and eventually extend beyond the intertriginous area. Secondary infection with *Candida albicans* in the intertriginous areas presents with small satellite pustules surrounding the red plaque. Mycological and/or bacteriological tests should distinguish these infective problems from psoriasis.

NAILS

The differential diagnosis depends on the type of nail lesions. Pitting of the nails without associated skin lesions around the nails is usually due to psoriasis. However, in *eczema* and *lichen planus*, pits have been described but there is skin involvement around the nails. Pits in nails have also been described in alopecia areata but hair loss is invariably present to elucidate the cause.

Onycholysis, when it occurs without psoriatic skin lesions, is sometimes referred to as idiopathic. It is more common on the finger nails, and in females. It is difficult to know whether idiopathic onycholysis is a separate entity or is due to underlying psoriasis. Onycholysis of the big toe nails may be due to trauma from foot wear. Onycholysis with subungual hyperkeratoses occurs in fungal infections, and mycology tests will be necessary to distinguish between psoriasis and a fungal infection.

Subungual hyperkeratosis with dystrophy of the nail plate is more common in psoriasis of the toe nails than the finger nails, and has to be distinguished from *fungal infections* by mycology tests.

Green discoloration under the nail plates is seen with onycholysis, whether idiopathic or due to psoriasis. A greenish-brown discoloration may be seen, but usually at the sides of the nails in dystrophy secondary to chronic candidal paronychia. The chronic paronychia suggests the diagnosis of candida.

Pustulation around the nail seen in some forms of acral psoriasis may also occur in *chronic paronychia*, whether it be candidal or bacterial. Red scaly patches around the nail support the diagnosis of psoriasis, and the appropriate pathological tests should also be carried out.

Splinter hemorrhages under the nail, which may be seen in psoriasis, also occur in *fungal infections, minor trauma, connective tissue diseases and subacute bacterial endocarditis*. The history and other clinical features should help to establish the appropriate diagnosis.

LINEAR PSORIASIS

Linear psoriasis (which is very rare) has to be distinguished from *linear nevi, lichen striatus* (linear eczema) and *linear lichen planus*. The clinical appearance should suggest the diagnosis. If not, a biopsy should be performed.

9

Psoriatic arthropathy

An association between psoriasis and arthritis was mentioned in the early part of the nineteenth century. However, there was no uniform agreement as to whether the arthropathy was part of the spectrum of rheumatoid arthritis or a separate entity. It is only in the past two or three decades that psoriatic arthropathy has been recognized as a separate disorder from rheumatoid arthritis. One of the problems in defining psoriatic arthropathy is whether it may exist without the skin lesions.

If this is accepted, then there appears to be significant overlap with ankylosing spondylitis and other spondarthritides. A working definition of psoriatic arthropathy would be 'an inflammatory arthritis, either peripheral or with spinal involvement, in association with psoriasis, and seronegative for the rheumatoid factor'.

EPIDEMIOLOGY

The incidence of arthropathy in patients with psoriasis has varied from 0.5 to 40% in different studies. This variation probably depends on the criteria used to establish the presence of an arthropathy, or missing the minimal skin involvement which may occur in some individuals. Conversely, in a recent study of screening patients with psoriasis for evidence of arthropathy using radiographs, it was found that approximately 50% had arthropathy[40]. However, in a large proportion, the individuals were symptomless and therefore, these patients would have been labeled as having no arthropathy.

Investigation of the incidence of psoriasis in patients with arthritis has shown a normal incidence for the seropositive, but an incidence four times the normal incidence in patients with seronegative arthritis, supporting the association between psoriasis and arthropathy. The overall incidence of psoriatic arthropathy in the general population has been estimated to be between 0.02 and 0.10%. The male : female sex ratio for psoriatic arthropathy has been shown to be 1 : 1.39, compared to 1 : 3 for rheumatoid arthritis. However, as mentioned above, these figures are based on arthropathy giving rise to symptoms, whilst occult changes in the joints are frequent in patients with psoriasis.

GENETICS

As with skin lesions, there is evidence to support a genetic mechanism in psoriatic arthropathy. Family studies have shown clustering, but no clear Mendelian pattern of inheritance has emerged. It appears that genetic transmission, as for the skin lesions, is based on multifactorial inheritance, with environmental factors playing an important part in triggering arthritis.

An increased incidence of HLA-B27 (95%) is now recognized in ankylosing spondylitis. This antigen has also been found to be raised in psoriatic arthritis if there is spinal involvement, the incidence being 80% for spinal involvement but 20% for peripheral arthritis. Other HLA antigens, A26, B38 and DR4, have been found to be raised in peripheral arthropathy. A recent study from Iceland has reported linkage to chromosome 16q for psoriatic arthritis. The study also found evidence for imprinting, showing a greater effect of paternal transmission[41].

CLINICAL FEATURES IN PERIPHERAL ARTHROPATHY

There are five groups of psoriatic arthropathy that have been outlined.

(1) The most common presentation is mono- or asymmetrical oligoarthropathy. This usually affects the interphalangeal joints, either the distal or proximal (Figures 109–111).

(2) Exclusive involvement of the distal interphalangeal joints of the toes or fingers. Involvement of these joints is said to be characteristic of psoriatic arthropathy, and distinguishes it from rheumatoid arthritis, which does not affect these joints.

(3) The presentation which is indistinguishable from rheumatoid arthritis, but the psoriatic disease runs a more benign course.

(4) A severe mutilating arthritis, as seen in rheumatoid disease, but with involvement of the distal interphalangeal joints.

(5) A peripheral arthropathy associated with sacroiliitis and/or spondylitis.

The incidence of the common oligoarthropathy has been found to be 50% of the psoriatic arthropathies. The severe mutilating form and localization to the distal interphalangeal joints have an incidence of 8% each.

Of all psoriatic patients with arthropathy, 30% have spondylitis.

The peak age of onset for psoriatic arthropathy is between 35 and 45 years. The severe mutilating form usually begins earlier. The onset is acute in approximately 50% of patients. The skin and joint lesions do not usually commence at the same time, but nail dystrophy and joint involvement often appear together.

SPINAL ARTHRITIS

There is now a recognized association between psoriasis and sacroiliitis and/or ankylosing spondylitis. The arthropathy may involve the sacroiliac joints and spine, together or separately. It is more common for both to be involved.

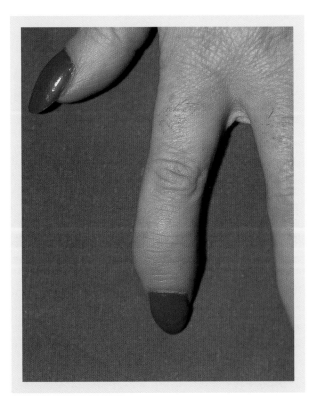

Figure 109 Involvement of the terminal interphalangeal joint in psoriatic arthritis. This is not seen in rheumatoid arthritis

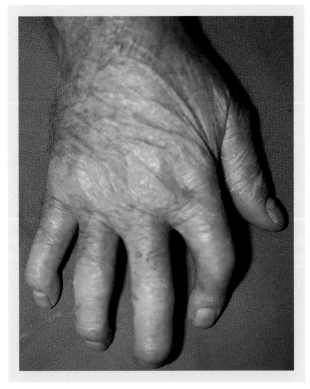

Figure 110 Psoriatic arthritis of the hand, involving both the proximal and the distal interphalangeal joints. The latter is characteristic of psoriatic arthropathy

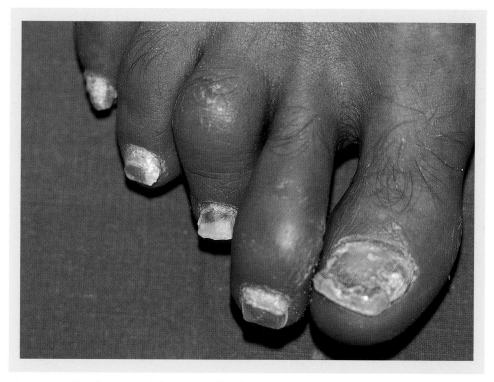

Figure 111 Involvement of the proximal and distal interphalangeal joints of the toes

RELATIONSHIP BETWEEN SKIN LESIONS AND ARTHROPATHY

The skin lesions appear first in the majority of patients, only 16% beginning with joint problems. In the latter group, those patients would be termed as having seronegative arthritis, until such time as they may develop the rash. It appears that there may be a small group with classical features of psoriatic arthropathy, i.e. distal interphalangeal involvement, who do not go on to develop psoriasis.

There is a strong association between generalized pustular psoriasis and arthritis; 30% of these patients have an arthropathy. It has been found in some surveys that the more extensive the psoriasis, the more likely the arthropathy.

RELATIONSHIP BETWEEN NAIL INVOLVEMENT AND ARTHROPATHY

There is a stronger association between joint involvement and nail abnormality than with skin lesions. It has been found that 85% of patients with arthropathy have nail involvement. The nail and joint problems often begin together. No particular one of the varying nail abnormalities is associated with the arthropathy.

EXTRA-ARTICULAR FEATURES

These have a lower incidence than those of rheumatoid arthritis. Subcutaneous nodules and involvement of the lung, heart or blood vessels do not occur. Ocular involvement has been reported, mainly uveitis and conjunctivitis. Episcleritis is rare.

Ankylosing spondylitis and inflammatory bowel disease have an increased incidence in patients with psoriatic arthritis.

TREATMENT

In its mildest forms no specific treatment is necessary. The drug therapy for the arthritis is the same as that for rheumatoid arthritis. NSAIDs will control a large proportion of patients. In a small number of patients, the NSAIDs appear to make the rash worse, but there is no way of predicting in which patient this may occur.

Other drugs that have been found to be helpful in severe disease are methotrexate, cyclosporin, azathioprine and gold salts. Methotrexate is the most effective of these drugs, and at a relatively low dose compared to that required to control the skin lesions. All have potential serious side-effects, and patients will have to be monitored closely. There are reports of improvement in the joints when the rash is treated with photo-chemotherapy (PUVA). Recently, monoclonal antibodies and fusion proteins directed against various cytokines and their receptors have been shown to be effective. These include: infliximab (antibody to TNFα) and etanercept (a recombinant TNFα receptor fusion protein), which binds to the TNFα receptor blocking, the effects of TNFα. These treatments are new and their exact role is yet to be defined. They are not without side-effects and there is no long-term data on their use in psoriatic arthritis.

Drugs to be avoided are antimalarials and systemic steroids. The former have been reported to make the rash worse, and with the latter there may be a flare-up of the rash when the dose of steroids is reduced.

Surgical procedures as for rheumatoid arthritis should be considered if there is severe deformity.

PROGNOSIS

The prognosis in psoriatic arthropathy appears to be better than in rheumatoid arthritis. There is generally less pain and disability. In a 10-year follow-up, one-third of the patients lost no time from work and 97% had less than 12 months' absenteeism. Radiologically, there is little deterioration in the majority of patients. Most of the reported fatalities in psoriatic arthropathy have been attributable to the drugs employed, but there is a small risk of amyloidosis.

10

Treatment

The management of psoriasis depends on the individual who is the patient. Only a small proportion of patients suffering from psoriasis present with symptoms requiring treatment, e.g. irritation in a small proportion; painful fissures, where there is involvement of the palms and soles and in the intertriginous areas; loss of mobility of the hands and feet with involvement at these sites; and systemic complications in erythrodermic and generalized pustular psoriasis. The main reason that patients seek treatment is because the disease is unsightly and therefore limits their social behavior.

When individuals first present with psoriasis, it is essential that the nature of the disease be explained to them. It is important that patients are told that psoriasis is not contagious and, in the mild and moderate forms, there are no serious complications. It should also be stressed that the exact cause of the disease is still to be elucidated but genetic factors are the basis of the disease and triggering factors such as stress, streptococcal infections, trauma to the skin and the drug lithium may initiate or aggravate psoriasis. The natural history should be explained and it must be emphasized that at present doctors cannot cure the disease, or even modify the course of the illness. Current treatments do not affect disease activity. If the disease is active, then relapse will occur as soon as treatment is discontinued, whatever therapy is used. The chance of remissions and their length do not depend on treatment. However, it is also important that patients are told that it is always possible to clear psoriasis with treatment currently available.

Many patients may choose not to treat their psoriasis when they realize the limitations of current therapeutic agents and are told of the benign nature of their disease. Other patients are unable to tolerate even minimal disease and demand treatment.

Most of the therapeutic agents used to treat psoriasis are based on empiricism or chance observations. It is only over the past few years that new therapies, based on scientific observation, have been tried. The current treatments can be divided into topical agents, those based on ultraviolet light, systemic drugs and so-called biologicals.

TOPICAL DRUGS

Topical drugs are: corticosteroids, coal tar, dithranol, vitamin D analogues, retinoids and immunosuppressives.

Topical corticosteroids

There is a good correlation between the potency of the steroid and its antipsoriatic action. Thus, the stronger the steroid the better it is at clearing psoriasis. Because of the wide variations in the potency of topical steroids, it is standard practice to divide them into four groups depending on their strength. The potency of a topical steroid is determined by biological assay (usually fibroblast inhibition or vasoconstriction). Hydrocortisone, which is the weakest topical steroid, is used as the standard with which to compare others.

Hydrocortisone (group I, a weak steroid) is designated to have 1 unit of steroid activity, moderate strength steroids (group II) 25 units, strong steroid 100 units (group III) and very strong, 600 units (group IV). Thus the range of steroid activity in those currently available is 1–600 units. It is important when prescribing topical steroids that the

Table I A selection of available topical corticosteroids

	Generic name	Trade name (UK)	Trade name (USA)
Group I (weak)	Hydrocortisone (0.5%, 1% and 2.5%)	Efcortelan	Cort-Dome
	Alclometasone dipropionate (0.05%)	Modrasone	Alcovate
Group II (intermediate strength)	Clobetasone butyrate (0.05%)	Eumovate	
	Hydrocortisone butyrate (0.1%)	Locoid	
	Flurandrenolone (0.0125%)	Haelan	
	Flurandrenolone acetonide (0.025%)		Cordran
Group III (strong)	Betamethasone valerate (0.1%)	Betnovate	Valisone
	Betamethasone (0.2%)		Celestone
	Fluocinolone acetonide (0.025%)	Synalar	Synalar
			Fluonid
	Halcinonide (0.1%)	Halciderm	Halog
	Fluocinonide (0.05%)	Metosyn	Lidex
	Beclomethasone dipropionate (0.025%)	Propaderm	–
	Fluocortolone pivalate (0.25%) +	Ultralanum	
	fluocortolone hexanoate (0.25%)		
	Flumethasone pivalate (0.03%)		Locorten
	Betamethasone dipropionate (0.05%)	Diprosone	Diprolene
	Diflucortolone valerate (0.1%)	Nerisone	
Group IV (very strong)	Clobetasol propionate (0.05%)	Dermovate	Temovate
	Fluocinolone acetonide (0.2%)		Synalar HP
	Diflucortolone valerate (0.3%)	Nerisone forte	

physician knows to which group the steroid belongs. Table 1 groups the majority of topical steroids in current use, depending on their potency.

Topical steroids can be applied as a lotion for scalp lesions, a cream for facial and intertriginous areas and an ointment for lesions on the trunk and limbs.

Advantages The main advantage of topical steroids is that they are pleasant to use. Group III and IV steroids are moderately effective in clearing chronic plaque psoriasis. Group II and III steroids can clear facial and intertriginous psoriasis. Group III and IV steroids in alcoholic solution are able to improve or sometimes clear lesions of the scalp.

Disadvantages One of the main disadvantages of topical steroids is that tachyphylaxis occurs when they are used for psoriasis. This means that the topical steroid will eventually lose its antipsoriatic effect. To maintain the clinical efficacy, the strength of the steroid will have to be increased and this increases the chance and incidence of side-effects. There is a limit to the strength of topical steroid available and, when this is reached, then topical steroids are no longer effective.

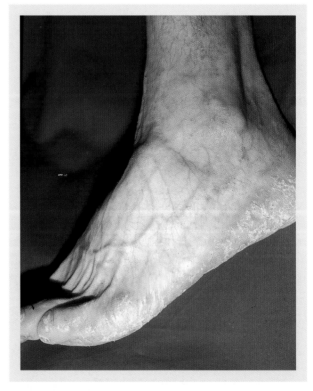

Figure 112 Thinning of the skin due to long-term use of potent, topical corticosteroids

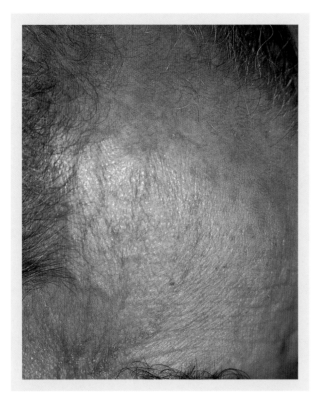

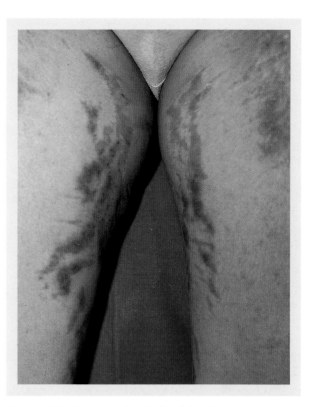

Figure 113 Telangiectasia of the upper forehead following long-term use of a potent, topical steroid scalp lotion

Figure 114 Striae on the thighs, following long-term use of a very potent topical steroid

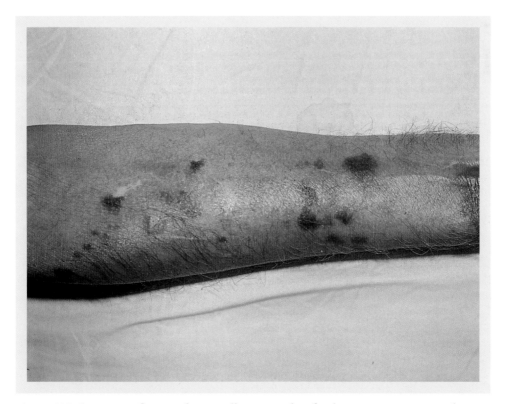

Figure 115 Purpura on forearm due to collagen atrophy after long-term potent steroids

Side-effects These are proportional to the strength of steroid and duration of use. In addition, side-effects are more commonly seen in intertriginous areas because of the greater absorption of the drug at these sites, due to the moist environment; and the face, where the skin is relatively thin. The local side-effects are due to collagen atrophy and inhibition of fibroblasts, and clinically these present as thin skin (Figure 112), telangiectasia (Figure 113), striae (Figure 114) and spontaneous bruising and purpura (Figure 115). Suppression of the pituitary adrenal axis and possibly cushingoid features only occur with group IV (and very occasionally group III) steroids. Topical steroids have to be used over long periods to produce these side-effects. As a general rule, 50 g of a group IV and 300 g of a group III steroid will have to be applied in a week to cause suppression of the pituitary adrenal axis.

Very occasionally, there can be a flare-up of the psoriasis when the topical steroid treatment is discontinued. This is usually only seen after the use of group IV steroids. The plaque may become pustular and enlarge. This rebound phenomenon may settle by itself; if not, weaker topical steroids (group II or III) may help. If the lesions are numerous and become more extensive, then one of the systemic drugs may have to be used.

In the past, topical steroids were used under polythene occlusion dressings to increase their efficacy. These dressings should not be used, as they will also increase the incidence and severity of side-effects.

Indications Group II and III topical steroids (in a cream base) are indicated for intertriginous and facial psoriasis.

Group III and IV steroids in an alcoholic lotion may be used on the scalp, if other preparations are not effective or tolerated.

Group III and IV steroids may be used for plaque psoriasis on the trunk and limbs. They should only be used as short courses, i.e. 2–3 weeks, and then stopped. If used for long periods, tachyphylaxis will occur and over long periods thinning of the surrounding skin may ensue.

Group II and III steroids are sometimes helpful in enhancing the resolution of guttate psoriasis.

Efficacy Topical steroids are moderately effective in the treatment of psoriasis.

Coal tar preparations

Coal tar preparations are the oldest substances still employed in the treatment of psoriasis, although they are being used less frequently. Crude coal tar is a mixture of approximately 10 000 compounds. Purification of the crude coal tar by distillation produces other mixtures which are pleasanter to use, but less efficacious. The mechanism of action of coal tar in psoriasis is unknown.

Preparations Crude coal tar is usually made up in an ointment base or as a paste. The concentration is usually 5–10%. Crude coal tar is often combined with salicylic acid 2–5%, which by its keratolytic action leads to better absorption of the coal tar.

Crude coal tar is used to treat only chronic plaque psoriasis and is usually combined with ultraviolet light.

Liquid coal tar is used in a variety of preparations for psoriasis. It is more acceptable to patients than crude coal tar. It is combined with keratolytics for use as a scalp preparation (10% liquid coal tar, 5% salicylic acid, 5% sulfur, 40% coconut oil, 40% emulsifying ointment). This particular preparation is usually applied at night and shampooed out the next morning. Liquid coal tar is frequently added to the bath water, either undiluted or in proprietary preparations.

Purified coal tar is added to shampoos, but has very little effect on scalp psoriasis.

Purified coal tar preparations are also used in cream and ointment bases for chronic plaque psoriasis, but, although they are cosmetically acceptable to the patient, their efficacy is poor.

Advantages Coal tar products are relatively safe and have very few side-effects.

Disadvantages Occasionally patients become sensitive to the coal tar and develop allergic reactions. A folliculitis may occur after the use of coal tar. The main disadvantage is the smell of crude coal tar. It is also unpleasant to use as it stains the clothes and bed clothes and the preparation has to be applied under tube gauze dressings. This makes it difficult to use as an outpatient unless the patient attends a special day center, which has its own drawback in that it is time-consuming, the patient having to attend hospital each day.

Efficacy This is relatively low compared to other drugs available for the treatment of psoriasis. The purified coal tar products are less efficacious than the unpurified coal tar preparations.

Indications For plaque psoriasis crude coal tar is used as a paste or ointment, or purified coal tar in a cream or ointment base. Liquid coal tar can be added to the bath water. For scalp psoriasis liquid coal tar is used, combined with keratolytics, and coal tar shampoos. *Contraindications* Coal tar products should not be used in the acute forms of psoriasis, i.e. guttate, erythrodermic or pustular psoriasis, as they may aggravate these conditions.

Dithranol

Dithranol, 1,8-dihydroxy-9-anthrone, is a naturally occurring substance found in the bark of the aroroba tree in South America. It can also be synthesized from anthrone. Its antipsoriatic action was noted over 100 years ago, when an extract of aroroba bark was used to treat psoriasis. The mechanism of action of dithranol in the treatment of psoriasis is still speculative.

Preparations Dithranol is made up in either a cream, ointment or paste. The advantage of using dithranol in a paste is that it is less likely to spread on to the surrounding skin. The disadvantage of using a paste is that it is difficult to remove.

There are two ways of using dithranol, either as an application over a 24-hour period, or as an application for only 15–30 minutes (short-contact dithranol). When used for 24 hours it is advisable to start

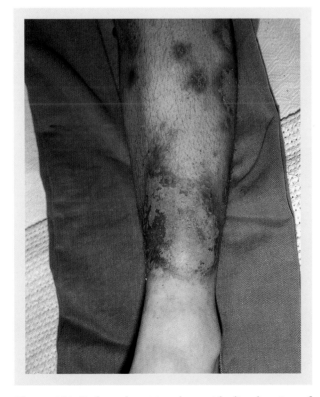

Figure 116 Dithranol staining: brownish discoloration of skin treated for a psoriatic plaque

with a concentration of 0.1%; if there is no burning or soreness then the concentration is gradually increased, usually every 3–4 days, to a maximum of 1.0%. It usually takes 3–4 weeks to clear psoriasis with dithranol. When used as a short-contact treatment, the initial concentration of dithranol is usually 2% and this may be increased to a maximum of 4%. The time taken to clear psoriasis with short-contact treatment is approximately the same as for the 24-hour treatment.

Short-contact treatment is usually given on an outpatient basis. It is imperative that the patient complies with the instructions, otherwise side-effects will occur. Short-contact treatment should not be recommended if compliance is in doubt.

Advantages Dithranol is probably the most effective topical antipsoriatic preparation currently available.

Disadvantages There are two main problems with dithranol treatment. First, dithranol stains the skin surrounding psoriatic plaques (Figure 116), the clothes, bed clothes, furniture and the bath a purple-brown color. Patients must be warned about this problem and dithranol must be used under tube gauze dressings. Patients should wear old pajamas when the drug is applied for 24 hours. When used for short-contact therapy, patients must wear old pajamas or clothes that they do not mind staining. The staining of the skin lasts up to 2 weeks after the dithranol is discontinued. It is difficult to remove the stains from clothing, bed clothes and furniture. The stains can be removed from the bath with either potassium permanganate or the detergent Teepol. The second problem with dithranol is that it causes an inflammatory reaction on the surrounding non-lesional skin. In its mildest form it is simply erythema; in its more severe forms it produces blisters (Figure 117) and erosions. This inflammatory reaction is accompanied by a burning sensation. If it is severe, the dithranol treatment has to be discontinued. Because of the inflammatory reaction to dithranol on non-lesional skin, dithranol should not be used in the intertriginous areas, on the face or near mucous membranes. If dithranol gets in the eyes, it can cause a severe inflammatory reaction with subsequent scarring of the conjunctivae.

Efficacy This is high, if the dithranol can be tolerated.

Indications Dithranol should only be used for chronic plaque psoriasis on the limbs and trunk.

Contraindications It should not be used for guttate, erythrodermic or pustular psoriasis.

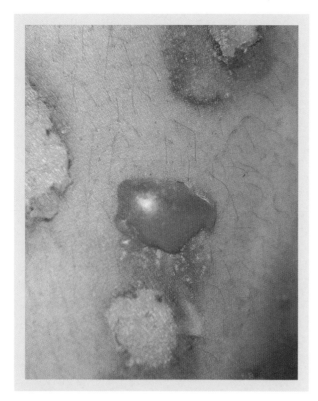

Figure 117 Blisters, due to dithranol, on uninvolved skin surrounding a psoriatic plaque

Vitamin D analogues

There are three vitamin D analogues currently being used as topical agents in psoriasis: calcipotriol, calcitriol and tacalcitol. The concept for their use in psoriasis is that they have the beneficial effect of vitamin D on psoriasis but with a considerably lower effect on calcium metabolism.

There are two postulated mechanisms for the beneficial effects of vitamin D analogues. First, vitamin D enhances differentiation of epithelial cells in psoriasis; there is a lack of differentiation of the keratinocytes. Second, vitamin D is said to have an inhibitory effect on CD4 T cells.

Preparations Calcipotriol is available as a cream, ointment or scalp lotion; whilst tacalcitol and calcitriol are only available in ointment bases.

Advantages Like topical steroids, they are pleasant to use.

Disadvantages These substances may cause irritation and irritant eczematous rash, particularly when applied to the face, and therefore should probably not be used at this site.

There is a limit to the amount that these preparations can be used; otherwise, they may affect calcium metabolism. The maximum recommended quantities per day for adults for the currently available preparations are calcipotriol 15 g; tacalcitol 10 g and calcitriol 30 g.

Efficacy Unfortunately, the efficacy for such a safe and pleasant to use preparations is relatively poor. There appears to be a small proportion of patients (about 25%) in which there is good efficacy.

Indications Vitamin D analogues are mainly indicated in stable chronic plaque psoriasis on the trunk and limbs. The calcipotriol scalp preparation is sometimes effective for stable disease.

Retinoids

The retinoid that is in current use for topical treatment is tazarotene.

Preparations Tazarotene is available in a gel at two strengths: 0.01% and 0.05%.

Advantages Because of the low concentrations used, no systemic effects have been recorded. No tachyphylaxis has been noted.

Disadvantages Local side-effects of burning, irritation and redness have been noted.

Efficacy This is only moderate. Improvement occurs, but total clearance is uncommon.

Indications Chronic plaque psoriasis on the trunk.

Contraindications Tazarotene should not be used on the face or intertriginous areas. It should not be used in pregnancy.

Topical calcineurin inhibitors

The two calcineurin inhibitors that are available for topical use are tacrolimus and pimecrolimus. Both are immunosuppressive as they inhibit cytokine production by activated T cells.

The topical preparations are helpful in some forms of atopic eczema but have been shown not to be effective in chronic plaque psoriasis. This is probably due to failure of penetration through the thick psoriatic scales. However, the preparations have been effective in facial (seborrheic) and intertriginous psoriasis. This is most likely to be due to ease of penetration through the relatively thin keratin layer in these types of psoriasis.

Preparations Tacrolimus is available in an ointment base at concentrations of 0.03% and 0.1%. Pimecrolimus is in an ointment base at a concentration of 1%.

Advantages These drugs do not cause thinning of the skin and, therefore, can be used on the face and intertriginous areas.

Disadvantages Both topical tacrolimus and pimecrolimus may cause a stinging or burning sensation. As they are immunosuppressive agents, they may increase the risk of skin malignancies, particularly if used long term on sun-exposed areas such as the face. Topical tacrolimus has been shown to accelerate carcinogenesis in animals[42].

Efficacy Moderate for facial and intertriginous psoriasis.

Indications Facial and intertriginous psoriasis not responsive to weak or moderate strength topical steroids at these sites.

Contraindications These preparations should not be used if viral, bacterial, or fungal infections are suspected. They should not be used on the face if there is a history of skin cancer or if there has been excessive exposure to strong sunlight, for example in Caucasians who have lived for long periods in warm, sunny climates.

ULTRAVIOLET LIGHT

It has been known for over 100 years that sunlight benefits psoriasis, and ultraviolet light has been used for treatment for 70 years. Ultraviolet light from artificial sources may be used by itself (phototherapy) or combined with drugs (photochemotherapy). Ultraviolet light can be divided into short wave (UVC 250–290 nm), middle wave (UVB 290–320 nm) and long wave (UVA 320–400 nm). UVC does not penetrate the earth's atmosphere, and benefit from sunlight is therefore from the UVB and UVA. The erythema and 'sunburn' effect of ultraviolet light is produced mainly by UVB. It requires a 1000 times greater dose for UVA to produce a similar effect. However, UVA intensity at the solar zenith is 100 times greater than UVB, and persists for much more of the day, so its effects in sunlight are not minimal. The main limiting factor of using ultraviolet light as a treatment for psoriasis is the 'sunburn' reaction. The paler the skin the more likely the patients are to 'burn'. This limits the amount of light they can receive, meaning the treatment is less effective. Patients can be divided into groups depending on their skin color, their ability to withstand the burning effect of ultraviolet light and their ability to tan. This classification is helpful in predicting the suitability of a particular patient for ultraviolet light treatment:

Group 1 – always burn, never tan

Group 2 – always burn, sometimes tan

Group 3 – sometimes burn, always tan

Group 4 – never burn, always tan

Group 5 – yellow-brown races

Group 6 – blacks

Phototherapy

This is now performed by so-called narrow-band UVB lamps. Although UVB is 290–320 nm, it has been shown that the anti-psoriatic effect is concentrated around 311 nm and lamps are now made that predominately emit this wavelength. These lamps also emit high-intensity 311 nm so that the duration of treatment is relatively short, and they are far more effective then the old broadband UVB lamps emitting rays of 290–320 nm.

Treatment with narrow-band UVB lamps is usually carried out three times per week with especially designed apparatus so that, if required, the whole body may be irradiated. Patients have to wear protective goggles during treatment.

Advantages The main advantage of UVB treatment is that no topical ointments, creams or oral medication are necessary. Patients with longstanding psoriasis find it a relief not to have to apply messy creams and ointments.

Disadvantages One of the principal disadvantages is that patients have to attend hospital on a regular basis for their treatment. If they do not live near the hospital, then it becomes a very time-consuming exercise or even an impossibility. UVB lamps for home use are available, but they are expensive.

With UVB irradiation alone, the clinical improvement is slow and it may take 8 weeks to clear or achieve significant improvement of psoriasis.

The only immediate potential side-effect is possible burning of the skin, if the dose is too high for that particular individual.

The long-term hazard of UVB treatment is its possible carcinogenic effect. There is some circumstantial evidence that basal and squamous cell carcinomas are due to chronic exposure to ultraviolet light, whilst melanoma may be induced by an acute sunburn reaction. Therefore, care must be taken not to burn patients. The treatment should not be continued indefinitely.

Efficacy Narrow-band UVB is effective in clearing chronic plaque psoriasis. However, it takes a relatively long time and is slower that photochemotherapy.

Indications Phototherapy is indicated for chronic plaque psoriasis not responsive to topical measures. It is not effective for scalp or intertriginous psoriasis because the UVB rays do not reach these sites. Phototherapy is sometimes used for guttate psoriasis to speed resolution.

Contraindications UVB should not be used for erythrodermic or generalized pustular psoriasis.

Laser

It has recently been shown that an excimer laser emitting 308 nm is effective in clearing resistant plaques of psoriasis.

Photochemotherapy (PUVA)

This treatment is based on the photosensitizing chemicals, psoralens. These occur naturally in plants but can also be synthesized. Psoralens exert their photosensitizing effect by absorbing light and then releasing this energy within the skin to exert biological effects. Psoralens also have the ability to combine with DNA in the presence of ultraviolet light. This was thought to be the basis of its action in psoriasis, as it would lead to inhibition of mitoses of the epidermal cells and hence proliferation. However, ultraviolet light also inhibits the function of APCs and lymphocytes and this effect is increased in the presence of psoralens.

The basis for PUVA (psoralens + UVA) treatment was the observation that UVA is 1000 times less likely to induce erythema and burning of the skin compared to UVB. It was suggested that, if only UVA was used, the psoralens would still exert their antiproliferative action, and yet 'burning' would be avoided. In practice, the combination of psoralens and UVA has proved to be a highly effective treatment for psoriasis.

Patients have to take the psoralens 2 hours before the UVA irradiation. The dose depends on body weight. The psoralen preparation usually used is 8-methoxy-psoralen. The dose is 20 mg if the body weight is under 50 kg, 30 mg if 51–65 kg, 40 mg if 66–80 kg, and 50 mg if over 80 kg. The treatment is carried out 2–3 times per week. The amount of UVA given initially depends on the skin type, and patients can be tested before treatment to determine the appropriate starting dose. The amount of UVA (measured in joules) is gradually increased to achieve satisfactory clearance of the psoriasis without inducing side-effects. Patients have to wear protective spectacles after taking the psoralen tablets and for at least the next 6 hours, as the eyes will be more sensitive to natural ultraviolet light and UVA from fluorescent lamps.

There are various machines for giving UVA treatment depending on the site of the psoriasis. There are machines designed to treat the whole body, or only hands or feet or scalp. The lamps used emit only UVA and visible light.

Advantages PUVA therapy has the same advantages as phototherapy with UVB, but it is more effective and quicker to achieve clearance than UVB alone.

Disadvantages Regarding the immediate side-effects, one of the main problems with PUVA is that the psoralens may cause nausea. This can be lessened to some extent by taking the drugs with food, or giving metoclopramide with the psoralens. Changing the psoralen preparation to 5-methoxypsoralen may help to diminish the nausea. Erythema and burning may occur, and if so the dose of UVA must be decreased. Pruritus is not an uncommon symptom, and pain may also be experienced. The pain and pruritus may be transitory, or prolonged, i.e. for many weeks, even though the treatment is discontinued. The cause of these symptoms is unknown but it has been suggested that it may be due to inflammation and damage to the nerve endings in the skin. A side-effect of PUVA, but one to which the patients do not usually object, is tanning.

The long-term side-effects include premature aging of the skin. If PUVA is continued as maintenance therapy or patients have repeated courses, then changes due to photoaging may be seen. These changes will depend on the amount of joules and the skin type. Lentigos are the commonest feature (Figure 118), but thinning and dryness of the skin also occur. Damage to the elastic tissue leads eventually to wrinkling.

Long-term PUVA treatment has been shown to be associated with an increase in squamous cell carcinomas. There is a strong dose–response relationship and the risk of developing these lesions continues after cessation of treatment[43]. Another feature was the high incidence on non-sun-exposed skin, e.g. male genitalia.

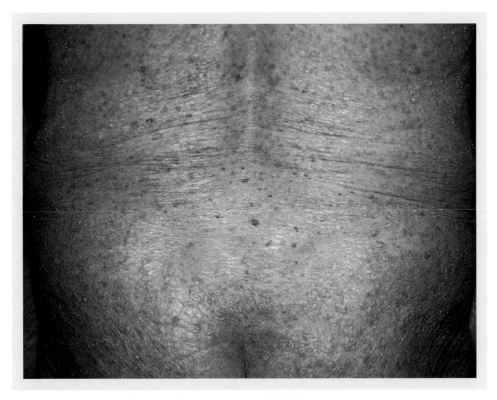

Figure 118 Numerous lentigos due to long-term PUVA for severe psoriasis

In contrast to squamous cell carcinoma, there has been only a modest increase in basal cell carcinomata and these have been on the trunk[43]. The risk of melanoma appears to be relatively low. There has been one report suggesting a possible increased risk[44].

To decrease the risk of malignancy, it has been recommended that the following measures be observed for both phototherapy and PUVA: protection of the male genitalia; protection of the face unless there is significant psoriasis; use of opaque protection for the lips; and use of protective eye wear.

Women who are pregnant or are contemplating pregnancy should not receive PUVA.

As with phototherapy, PUVA is not effective for scalp or intertriginous psoriasis, as the UVA does not reach these areas.

Efficacy PUVA is a very effective treatment for psoriasis, and approximately 95% of patients who can tolerate the treatment will have good results. Nausea and pruritus are the main limiting factors.

Indications PUVA is indicated for chronic plaque disease which is extensive or has failed to respond to topical treatment. It is also effective for localized pustular psoriasis of the palms and soles. It is effective in guttate psoriasis, but, because this condition is of short duration, PUVA is not usually indicated.

Contraindications PUVA, as a general rule, should not be used for erythrodermic or generalized pustular psoriasis.

Topical PUVA

Instead of taking psoralens by mouth, they can be applied directly to the skin. If the psoriasis is extensive then the psoralen solution is added to bath water and the patients soak in the bath for 20 minutes. Immediately after the immersion, the skin is dried and the skin exposed to the UVA irradiation. The main advantage of bath PUVA is that no oral medication is required and thus, there are no systemic side-effects such as nausea. The disadvantages are the extra time that the patient has to attend the treatment center and the extra space required for the bath.

For small areas of involvement such as the palms and soles, a cream containing psoralen can be applied to the affected areas and treated with UVA after 1 hour.

Climatic therapy

Many patients know that going to a sunny climate improves their psoriasis, but there are a small proportion of patients who find that their psoriasis may actually deteriorate in the sun. For those whose psoriasis improves, the nearer the equator the more potent the effects of the sunlight. Patients should be warned not to over-expose themselves in the first few days, as sunburn may actually progress to psoriasis (the Koebner phenomenon). It usually takes 4 weeks to clear psoriasis in an appropriate climate.

As already mentioned, one of the problems of self-treatment in the sunnier parts of the world is sunburn. This problem is overcome by going to the Dead Sea. This curious result is due to the unique geographical features of the Dead Sea. It is the deepest place on the Earth's surface and is surrounded by mountains. The sea evaporates and forms an aerosol which stays in the atmosphere above the sea and surrounding beaches. This aerosol screens out the majority of the UVB rays but not the UVA. This mixture of ultraviolet light at the earth's surface is sufficient to clear psoriasis but prevent sunburn. Thus patients can stay on the shores of the Dead Sea all day without risk of sunburn. It is also claimed that the chemicals in the Dead Sea speed the resolution of psoriasis. There is no doubt that the Dead Sea is more effective than other parts of the world in clearing psoriasis, but it still takes 4 weeks for this to happen. The only disadvantages of this treatment are time and expense.

ORAL THERAPY

The three most commonly used drugs are methotrexate, acitretin and cyclosporin. They are limited to severe disease as they all have potential serious side-effects. The drug chosen as the first line of systemic treatment is the personal choice of the physician.

Methotrexate

Methotrexate is a folic acid antagonist which has been used for psoriasis for the past 40 years. The beneficial effect on psoriasis was a chance observation when these drugs were being used for rheumatoid arthritis for a supposed anti-inflammatory effect. A number of patients with psoriatic arthritis were also included in the study, and it was noted that the psoriatic skin lesions cleared.

Methotrexate is given weekly. A test dose of 5.0 mg should be given and if there are no untoward side-effects, the dose can be increased. The dose to clear psoriasis varies between patients but is usually 10–30 mg weekly. Very occasionally, a higher dose may be necessary. The dose for a particular patient has to be found by altering the dose according to the clinical response.

Prior to initiating methotrexate, patients must have a full blood count, tests of liver function and serum creatinine, urine analysis and chest X-ray. Patients with abnormal liver or renal function should probably not be given methotrexate. Whether a liver biopsy is performed prior to initiating methotrexate is a matter of choice for the physician. Routine monitoring of full blood count and liver function are mandatory. The indications for liver biopsy have changed over the last few years. Originally it was advocated that liver biopsies were performed prior to initiation of treatment and then yearly. It is now considered unnecessary to perform liver biopsies on a yearly basis or prior to treatment. Monitoring of hepatotoxicity with routine liver function tests and the serum level of the amino-terminal propeptide of type III procollagen (PIIINP) are sufficient in the majority of patients. PIIINP is a measure of fibrogenesis and has been shown to correlate with methotrexate-induced fibrosis of the liver. It should be remembered that liver biopsy is not without morbidity and even mortality and the decision of perform a liver biopsy should be taken by a hepatologist familiar with methotrexate-induced hepatotoxicity.

Advantages Methotrexate is a highly effective drug in clearing psoriasis and maintaining the improvement.

Disadvantages Regarding the immediate side-effects, some patients experience nausea and lethargy for 24–48 hours after taking methotrexate. Oral and gastrointestinal ulceration and suppression of the bone marrow are the main immediate side-effects. Some patients appear to be sensitive to these side-effects and this is the reason for giving a small test dose prior to initiating treatment to clear psoriasis. Once the patient is established on a maintenance dose, the risk of ulceration of the alimentary tract and bone marrow suppression recedes.

The main long-term side-effect is damage to the liver. Methotrexate is hepatotoxic and there may be a slight rise in liver enzymes in the first few days after taking the drug. However, this hepatotoxicity may lead to fibrosis and eventually cirrhosis. The risk of serious liver damage is related to the cumulative dose and duration of treatment although as with most drugs there is patient variability to side-effects. Methotrexate has been shown to raise the blood homocysteine levels. Increased levels of homocysteine may promote atherosclerosis and subsequent thrombosis. It has been reported in rheumatoid arthritis patients treated with methotrexate that there is an increase in cardiovascular co-morbidity thought to be due to a raised homocyteine levels. This effect of methotrexate can be countered by giving patients folic acid 5 mg daily.

Efficacy Methotrexate is very effective in clearing psoriasis.

Indications Methotrexate is indicated for severe plaque psoriasis unresponsive to topical measures and ultraviolet light treatments, and erythrodermic and generalized pustular psoriasis.

Contraindications Methotrexate is contraindicated in pregnancy, severe impairment of hepatic or renal function, and if patients are receiving drugs which interact with methotrexate.

Acitretin

Acitretin is a retinoid. These are analogues of vitamin A and were developed primarily as anti-cancer agents. The observation that vitamin A deficiency is associated with follicular hyperkeratoses, dryness of the lips and general dryness of the skin led to the suggestion that some of the analogues of vitamin A may improve disorders associated with abnormal keratinization.

Of the vitamin A analogues available, acitretin has been found to be helpful in psoriasis. The dose is 0.5–1.0 mg/kg per day. When used as the sole treatment for plaque psoriasis, it may take up to 3 or 4 months before there is significant improvement. However, the beneficial effect on generalized pustular psoriasis is apparent within days.

Advantage As with other oral treatments, the simplicity of use is of considerable benefit to the patient.

Disadvantages Probably the most important side-effect of all retinoids is that they are teratogenic. Unfortunately, acitretin is not totally cleared from the body for 2 years after discontinuing the drug. Therefore, as a general rule, women of child-bearing age should not receive acitretin for psoriasis.

Immediate side-effects After approximately 2 weeks, patients develop dryness and peeling of the lips. In the more severe forms of cheilitis, there may be fissuring and secondary infection. Other mucous membranes may also be affected, particularly the nasal mucosa leading to epistaxis. Conjunctivitis is a rarer complication. The skin may become red and scaly and this is more common on the face. Another rare complication is swelling and redness of the nail folds, mimicking paronychia. Scaling of the scalp and diffuse thinning of the hair may also occur. All the side-effects are reversible when the acitretin is discontinued.

Long-term side-effects A rise in serum lipids occurs in nearly half of the patients taking long-term acitretin. This increase is reversible when the drug is discontinued. Hepatotoxicity is a rare complication. Extraosseous ossification may occur around joints. The true incidence of this complication is not known, because radiographs are not routinely taken during therapy.

Efficacy The beneficial effect of acitretin is variable between patients. A major drawback is that it is slower than methotrexate and cyclosporin in clearing psoriasis.

Indications Acitretin is indicated for severe plaque psoriasis unresponsive to topical measures and ultraviolet light treatments, and generalized pustular psoriasis.

Contraindications Acitretin is contraindicated in hyperlipidemia and impaired liver function, and should not be used by pregnant women, or ideally in women of child-bearing age.

Cyclosporin

Cyclosporin has been used for psoriasis for the past 20 years. It was used intentionally because of the known action of cyclosporin in inhibiting activated CD4 (T helper) lymphocytes, which are central to the pathogenesis of psoriasis.

The initial dose of cyclosporin for psoriasis should be 3 mg/kg per day. If there is no significant improvement after 2 weeks, the dose may be increased to 4 mg/kg per day. If there is no improvement after a further 2 weeks, the dose may be increased to 5 mg/kg per day. However, this latter dose should not be exceeded, because there is an increased risk of side-effects. A small proportion of patients are able to control their psoriasis with a daily dose of 1–2 mg/kg. The dose may vary from time to time in an individual depending on the activity of the disease.

Prior to treatment with cyclosporin, it is mandatory to ensure that patients have normal renal function. Serum creatinine and urine analysis may not be sensitive enough to identify early renal damage, and therefore, ideally, the glomerular filtration rate should be determined before initiating treatment. A full blood count and liver function tests should also be performed before starting treatment. The blood pressure must also be taken before beginning treatment.

During treatment, regular monitoring (approximately every 4–6 weeks) of blood pressure, serum creatinine and liver function is necessary. If long-term treatment is undertaken, then the glomerular filtration rate should be determined annually. A small decrease of the glomerular filtration rate is to be expected, but, if it is greater than 35%, then cyclosporin should probably be discontinued. A rise in serum creatinine greater than 30% of the baseline value also implies significant impairment of renal function and it is advisable to try to control the psoriasis with a lower dose if possible. If the serum creatinine rises to more than 50% of the baseline value, then cyclosporin should be discontinued.

Because there is a relatively good correlation between renal function (as measured by the glomerular filtration rate) and renal biopsy findings during long-term cyclosporin treatment, it is probably not necessary to perform routine renal biopsies. However, if cyclosporin has to be continued because of the severity of the psoriasis and inability to control the disease with other drugs, then renal biopsy should probably be performed if the renal function tests imply a significant decrease in function, so that an accurate assessment of nephrotoxicity can be made.

Advantages Cyclosporin is a highly effective treatment for psoriasis. It has fewer subjective side-effects than methotrexate and acitretin and is, therefore, preferred by the patients.

Disadvantages The minor side-effects that patients may experience are nausea, paraesthesia and hypertrichosis. However, these are usually not severe and do not require cessation of therapy. The two main problems associated with cyclosporin are hypertension and nephrotoxicity. There are two clinical patterns of hypertension associated with cyclosporin. In the first, the hypertension develops within the first 3 months of starting treatment and the inci-

dence is approximately 15%. In the second pattern, hypertension develops after long-term treatment, i.e. after 2 years or more. The incidence of hypertension developing late in treatment is related to duration of therapy. Thus, after 2 years, the incidence is approximately 30% and at 5 years 40%. Fortunately, the hypertension associated with cyclosporin is not severe, and can be controlled with hypotensive agents. The calcium channel blocker nifedipine is the most suitable drug with which to initiate hypotensive treatment. The hypertension due to cyclosporin is reversible when the drug is discontinued.

The second problem associated with cyclosporin is nephrotoxicity. Cyclosporin causes constriction of the renal arterioles and thus there may be an immediate but small decrease in renal function. If cyclosporin is continued for long periods, there may be structural changes in the kidney, consisting of tubular atrophy, increased interstitial fibrosis, hyaline deposits in the renal arterioles and an increase in glomerular obsolescence. Severe renal damage should be preventable by close monitoring of patients and cessation of therapy if necessary.

All patients who are immunosuppressed run a risk of increased malignancy and, therefore, this is a potential hazard with cyclosporin treatment. Indeed, a recent study has shown a six-fold higher incidence of skin malignancies in patients taking cyclosporin for more than 2 years[45]. Most of the malignancies were squamous cell carcinomas. There was no increase in melanomas or non-skin malignancies but close follow-up of patients taking cyclosporin for longer periods is necessary.

Efficacy Cyclosporin is a very effective drug for clearing psoriasis.

Indications Cyclosporin should be reserved for severe chronic plaque disease (unresponsive to topical measures and ultraviolet light treatments), erythrodermic, localized pustular psoriasis and generalized pustular psoriasis.

Contraindications Cyclosporin is contraindicated in patients with impaired renal function, malignancy and chronic infections.

Rotation of systemic drugs

As psoriasis is a chronic disease, particularly when severe, treatment may have to be continued indefinitely in some individuals. To decrease the incidence and severity of nephrotoxicity and hypertension associated with cyclosporin and the hepatotoxicity of methotrexate, it may be advisable to rotate the use of these two effective treatments. Rotating the drugs every 6 months may diminish the side-effects.

Other systemic drugs

Both hydroxyurea and azathioprine have been used in the past. However, azathioprine is not very effective, and, although hydroxyurea has a better therapeutic effect, it is not as good as methotrexate or cyclosporin. In addition, hydroxyurea frequently causes bone marrow suppression.

Mycophenolate mofetil has also been used for psoriasis. It has been shown to be effective but less so than cyclosporin[46]. The main side-effects are gastrointestinal, usually diarrhea, and bone marrow suppression.

Systemic steroids should not, as a general rule, be used for psoriasis. There is always a risk of 'rebound' when the steroids are reduced. Systemic steroids have been used in high dosage (e.g. 100 mg prednisolone daily) for erythrodermic psoriasis, but cyclosporin or methotrexate are now usually preferred.

Recently systemic pimecrolimus, which is a calcineurin inhibitor, has been shown to be effective in clearing psoriasis[47]. It has a similar mechanism of action to cyclosporin and inhibits cytokine production by T cells. However, unlike cyclosporin it does not appear to be nephrotoxic.

COMBINED TREATMENTS

Therapeutic agents for psoriasis are often combined; first, because they may have a synergistic effect, and second, to decrease the side-effects of one, or both, of the treatments.

Topical corticosteroids and vitamin D analogues

It has been shown that topical corticosteroids and vitamin D analogues have a synergistic action. Thus, a better response is obtained and less topical steroid is required to achieve a satisfactory clinical response.

Coal tar and ultraviolet light

This combination has been used for many years and enhances the speed of clearance compared to the individual modalities.

Acitretin and photochemotherapy

Acitretin has been shown to lower the amount of UVA in PUVA treatment necessary to clear psoriasis. However, even if acitretin is taken for only a few weeks, women of childbearing age have to avoid pregnancy for 2 years. Another drawback is that patients usually develop cheilitis and dryness of the skin.

Systemic drugs and topical treatment

Not infrequently, a few resistant plaques of psoriasis may remain when patients are treated with cyclosporin, methotrexate or acitretin. If these patches are a nuisance to the patient, it may be possible to clear them with the addition of topical steroids or vitamin D analogues rather than increasing the dose of the systemic drug.

A combination of the current systemic drugs is not advisable, because of the increased risk of side-effects.

BIOLOGICALS

The term 'biologicals' has been coined to denote treatments that are designed to alter an immune response or block a specific pathway in this response. Examples of those altering the response are recombinant human cytokines, whereas targeted treatments include fusion proteins and monoclonal antibodies. The various 'targets' chosen are based on the knowledge of the immunopathogenesis of psoriasis elucidated over the past 20 years. The targets chosen have included the trafficking of T cells from the blood vessels into the skin (Figure 13), antigen presentation from APCs to lymphocytes (Figure 8) and blocking of the action of cytokines.

Recombinant cytokines

IL-10 This cytokine has been shown to be inhibitory for a Th1 immune response. It has been suggested that IL-10 shifts the T cell response from Th1 to Th2. IL-10 has been used in trials for the treatment of psoriasis and shown to be reasonably effective, i.e. a reduction of 55% in the Psoriasis Area Severity Index (PASI)[48]. Recombinant IL-10 is reasonably well tolerated.

IL-4 This cytokine is characteristic of a Th2 immune response, associated with allergic or atopic disorders.

IL-4 down-regulates the production of IFNγ, which is characteristic of a Th1 response as seen in psoriasis. Treatment with IL-4 has been shown to improve psoriasis.

Anticytokines

TNFα plays an important role in the pathogenesis of psoriasis, so blocking its action should improve psoriasis.

Infliximab

Infliximab is a chimeric human TNFα monoclonal antibody derived from mice. It has to be given by infusion. The improvement in psoriasis may be seen within 2 weeks, and approximately 80% of patients show significant clearing of their skin lesions[49].

Inflixmab has a number of side-effects, including infusion reactions and reactivation of latent tuberculosis. Neutralizing antibodies develop to infliximab and make treatment less effective over time.

Etanercept

Etanercept is a recombinant TNFα receptor fusion protein, which will bind to TNFα and form a complex, so the cytokine is no longer available to perform its biological functions. Etanercept has been shown to be effective in psoriasis and the results are dose dependent. With low dose (25%), medium dose (44%) and high dose (59%), all showed significant improvement, i.e. a reduction in their psoriasis score of 75%. Etanercept has to be given by injection[50].

Side-effects can include reactions at the site of injection. Neutralizing antibodies have been found in some patients. Antinuclear antibodies and antibodies to double-stranded DNA in a few patients with systemic lupus erythematosus have been reported. Other serious side-effects, but with a low incidence, are aplastic anemia, demyelinating diseases and tuberculosis, probably due to reactivation of latent disease.

Alfacept

Alfacept is a fusion protein, which contains a binding site of LFA-3. Memory T cells, which play a role in the pathogenesis of psoriasis, express CD2, which is a ligand of LFA-3. The binding of LFA-3 to CD2 is one of the pathways for activation of T cells by APCs

and this is termed a co-stimulating signal (Figure 8). Alfacept binds to CD2 and stops T cell activation.

Alfacept has to be given by intramuscular injection or infusion like other 'biologicals'. Studies have shown reasonable results for alfacept with over half the treated patients achieving at least 50% reduction in their psoriasis score. Experience with alfacept is less than with etanercept and infliximab, and its safety profile has yet to be determined.

Efalizumab

Efalizumab is a humanized monoclonal antibody to CD11A, which is a component of LFA-1 present on the surface of T cells. LFA-1 binds to ICAM-1, which is found on APCs and endothelial cells. By blocking the bindings of LFA-1 on T cells to ICAM-1 on APCs (Figure 8), efalizumab inhibits activation of T cells. By blocking the binding LFA-1 on T cells and ICAM-1 on endothelial cells (Figure 13), it will prevent recruitment of T cells into the skin, which is an integral part of the pathogenesis of psoriasis.

Trials of efalizumab in the treatment of psoriasis have shown moderate results with 28% of patients achieving a reduction in the psoriasis score by more than 75% and 57% of patients by more than 50%. Side-effects were common and consisted of headaches, nausea and vomiting, fever and myalgia. These effects were transitory[51].

General comment on biologicals

The development of antibodies and fusion proteins to components of the immune pathways in psoriasis have been heralded by some as a major advance in the treatment of psoriasis. However, as yet, no pathway has been identified that is specific for psoriasis. The same pathways occur in other chronic inflammatory conditions such as rheumatoid arthritis and Crohn's disease and that is why the same agents used for psoriasis are also effective in these other diseases. The immune system has evolved over millions of years to protect the living animal against micro-organisms. It is also concerned with the emergence and course of malignant tumors. Thus, blocking various pathways of the immune response may have serious long-term effects. It is early days in the use of these agents for chronic inflammatory diseases such as psoriasis, and careful long-term follow-up of individuals receiving these treatments is necessary.

FUTURE TREATMENTS

These will depend on a greater understanding of the pathogenesis of psoriasis. The newer 'biologicals' which are now being used, were forecast in the first edition of this book, 12 years ago[52]. Genetic studies have not so far been rewarding but they may be in the future. Identification of the genes may allow development of therapeutic agents to block the proteins expressed by the genes. Identifying the antigen, if it is bacterial, may be more promising. Blocking the presentation of peptides to the immune cells or even vaccination may become treatments in the future.

References

1. Lomholt G. Psoriasis. Prevalence, Spontaneous Course and Genetics. Copenhagen: G.E.C. Gad, 1963

2. Fry L, McMinn RMH. The action of chemotherapeutic agents on psoriatic epidermis. *Br J Dermatol* 1968;80:373–83

3. Romanus T. Psoriasis from a prognostic and hereditary point of view. Dissertation, Uppsala, 1945

4. Farber EM, Nall ML. The natural history of psoriasis in 5000 patients. *Dermatologica* 1974;148:1–18

5. Enfors W, Molin L. Pustulosis palmaris et plantaris. *Acta Dermatol Venereol* 1971;51:289–94

6. Williams RC, McKenzie AW, Roger JH, Joysey VC. HL-A antigens in patients with guttate psoriasis. *Br J Dermatol* 1976;95:163–7

7. Martin BA, Chalmers RJG, Telfer N. How great is the risk of further psoriasis following a single episode of acute psoriasis? *Arch Dermatol* 1996;132:717

8. Hoede K. Ubersichten zur Frage der Erblichkeit der Psoriasis. *Hautzart* 1957;8:433–8

9. Hellgren L. *Psoriasis*. Stockholm: Almquist & Wiksell, 1967

10. Tiilikainen A, Lassus A, Karvonen J, et al. Psoriasis and HLA-Cw6. *Br J Dermatol* 1980;102:179–84

11. Ozawa A, Okkido M, Inoko H, et al. Specific restriction fragment length polymorphism on the HLA-C region and susceptibility to psoriasis. *J Invest Dermatol* 1988;90:402–5

12. Cao K, Song FJ, Li HG, et al. Association between HLA antigen and families with psoriasis vulgaris. *Chin Med J* 1993;106:132–5

13. Gudjonsson J, Karason A, Antonsdottir A, et al. Psoriasis patients who are homozygous for HLA – Cw6* 0602 allele have a 2.5-fold increased risk of developing psoriasis compared with Cw6 heterozygotes. *Br J Dermatol* 2003;148:233–5

14. Hensler T, Christopher E. Psoriasis of early and late onset: characteristics of two types of psoriasis. *J Am. Acad Dermatol* 1985;13:450–6

15. Gudjonsson J, Karason A, Antonsdottir A, et al. HLA-Cw6 positive and HLA-Cw6 negative patients with psoriasis vulgaris have distinct clinical features. *J Invest Dermatol* 2002;118:362–5

16. Tiwari JL, Lowe NJ, Abramovits W, et al. Association of psoriasis with HLA-DR7. *Br J Dermatol* 1982;106:227–30

17. Baker BS, Ovigne JM, Fischetti VA, et al. Reduced IFN gamma responses associated with HLA-DR15 presentation of streptococcal cell wall proteins to dermal Th-1 cells in psoriasis. *J Clin Immunol* 2003;23:407–14

18. Capon F, Munro M, Barker J, Trembeth R. Searching for the major histocompatibility complex psoriasis susceptibility gene. *J Invest Dermatol* 2002;118: 745–51

19. Traupe H. The complex genetics of psoriasis revisited. In Van de Kerkhof P, ed. *Textbook of Psoriasis*. Oxford: Blackwell Publishing, 2003:70–82

20. Helms C, Cao L, Krueger JG, et al. A putative RUNX 1 binding site variant between SLC9A3R1 and NAT9 is associated with susceptibility to psoriasis. *Nature Genet* 2003;35:349–56

21. Hewett D, Samuelsson L, Polding J, et al. Identification of a psoriasis susceptibility candidate gene by linkage disequilibrium mapping with a localised single nucleotide polymorphism map. *Genomics* 2002;79:305–14

22. Norholm-Pederson A. Infections and psoriasis. *Acta Dermatol Venereol* 1952;32:159–67

23. Belew PW, Wannamaker LW, Johnson D, Rosenberg EW. Beta haemolytic streptococcal types associated with psoriasis. In Kimura K, Kotami S, Shiokawa Y, eds. *Recent Advances of Streptococcal Diseases*. Reedbooks Ltd, 1985:334

24. Telfer NR, Chalmers RJ, Whale K, Coleman G. The role of streptococcal infection in the initiation of guttate psoriasis. *Arch Dermatol* 1992;128:39–42

25. Cohen Tervart WC, Esseveld H. A study of the incidence of haemolytic streptococci in the throat in patients with psoriasis with reference to their role in the pathogenesis of the disease. *Dermatologica* 1970;140:282–90

26. Wardrop P, Weller R, Marais J, *et al.* Tonsillitis and chronic psoriasis. *Clin Otolaryngol* 1998;23:67–8

27. Baker BS. B Haemolytic streptococci and psoriasis. In *Recent Advances in Psoriasis: The Role of the Immune System*. London: Imperial College Press, 2000:61–89

28. Leung DYM, Walsh P, Giorno R, Norris DA. A potential role for superantigens in the pathogenesis of psoriasis. *J Invest Dermatol* 1993;100:225–8

29. Baker BS, Powles AV, Garioch JJ, *et al.* Differential T cell reactivity to round and oval forms of *Pityrosporum* in the skin of patients with psoriasis. *Br J Dermatol* 1997;136:319–25

30. Valdimarsson H, Baker BS, Jonsdottir I, Fry L. Psoriasis, a disease of abnormal keratinocyte proliferation medicated by T cells. *Immunol Today* 1986;7:256–7

31. Gudjonsson JE, Johnston A, Sigmunsdottir H, *et al.* Immunopathogenic mechanisms in psoriasis. *Clin Exp Immunol* 2004;135:1–8

32. Lewis HM, Baker BS, Bokth S, *et al.* Restricted T cell receptor VB gene usage in the skin of patients with guttate and chronic plaque psoriasis. *Br J Dermatol* 1993;129:514–20

33. Leung DYM, Travers JB, Giorno R, *et al.* Evidence of streptococcal superantigens-driven process in acute guttate psoriasis. *J Clin Invest* 1995;96:2106–12

34. Sigmundsdottir H, Sigurgeirsson B, Troye-Blomberg M, *et al.* Circulating T cells of patients with active psoriasis respond to streptococcal M-peptides sharing sequences with human epidermal keratins. *Scand J Immunol* 1997;45:688–97

35. Gudmundsdottir AS, Sigmundsdottir H, Sigurgeirsson B, *et al.* Is an epitope on keratin 17 a major target for autoreactive T lymphocytes in psoriasis. *Clin Exp Immunol* 1999;117:580–6

36. Brown DW, Baker BS, Ovigne JM, et al. Non-M protein(s) on the cell wall and membrane of group A streptococci induce(s) IFNγ production by dermal CD4+ T cells on psoriasis. *Arch Dermatol Res* 2001;293:165–70

37. Baker BS, Brown DW, Fischetti VA, *et al.* Skin T cell proliferative responses to M protein and other cell wall and membrane proteins of group A streptococci in chronic plaque psoriasis. *Clin Exp Immunol* 2001;124:516–21

38. Chang JC, Smith LR, Froning KJ, *et al.* CD8+ T cells in psoriatic lesions preferentially use T cell receptor V beta 3 and/or VB 13.1 genes. *Proc Natl Acad Sci USA* 1994;91:9282–6

39. Nickoloff BJ, Wrone-Smith T. Injections of pre-psoriatic skin with CD4+ T cells induces psoriasis. *Am J Pathol* 1999; 155:145–58

40. Lewis JS, Raqvindran JS, Korendowych E, *et al.* Prevalence and characteristics of undiagnosed psoriatic arthropathy in psoriasis: a challenge for genetic studies. *Br J Dermatol* 2002;147:1052–3. (Abstr.)

41. Karason A, Gudjonsson JE, Upmanyu R, *et al.* A susceptibility gene for psoriatic arthritis maps to chromosome 16q: evidence for imprinting. *Am J Hum Genet* 2003;72:125–31

42. Niwa Y, Terashima T, Sumi H. Topical application of the immunosuppressant tacrolimus accelerates carcinogenesis in mouse skin. *Br J Dermatol* 2003; 149:960–7

43. Stern RS, Laird N. For the photochemotherapy follow-up study. The carcinogenic risk of treatments for severe psoriasis. *Cancer* 1994;73:2759–64

44. Stern RS, Nichols KT, Vakeva LH. Malignant melanoma in patients treated for psoriasis with methoxalen (psoralen) and ultraviolet light A irradiation (PUVA). *N Engl J Med* 1997;336:1041–5

45. Paul CF, Ho VC, McGeown C. Risk of malignancies in psoriasis patients treated with cyclosporine: a 5-year cohort study. *J Invest Dermatol* 2003; 120:211–16

46. Davison SC, Morris-Jones R, Powles AV, Fry L. Change of treatment from cyclosporine to mycophenolate mofetil in severe psoriasis. *Br J Dermatol* 2000;143:405–7

47. Rappersberg K, Komar M, Ebelin ME, *et al.* Pimecrolimus identifies a common genomic anti-inflammatory profile, is highly effective in psoriasis and is well tolerated. *J Invest Dermatol* 2002; 119:876–87

48. Assadullah K, Docke WD, Ebeling M, *et al.* Interleukin 10 treatment of psoriasis: clinical results in a phase II trial. *Arch Dermatol* 1999;135:187–92

49. Lebwohl M. Psoriasis. *Lancet* 2003;361:1197–204

50. Leonardi CL, Powers JL, Matheson RT, *et al.* Etanercept as monotherapy in patients with psoriasis. *N Engl J Med* 2003;349:2014–22

51. Lebwohl M, Tyring SK, Hamilton TK, *et al.* A novel targeted T cell modulator, efalizumab, for plaque psoriasis. *N Engl J Med* 2003;349:2004–13

52. Fry, L. *An Atlas of Psoriasis*. Carnforth, UK: Parthenon Publishing, 1992:51–2

Index